Special Topics in Biology Series

Comparative Physiology of Respiration

John D. Jones
B.Sc., Ph.D.
Senior Lecturer in Zoology, University of Sheffield

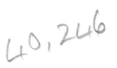

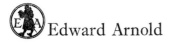Edward Arnold

First published 1972,
by Edward Arnold (Publishers) Ltd.,
41 Maddox Street,
London, W1R 0AN

Boards edition ISBN 0 7131 2339 7
Paper edition   ISBN 0 7131 2340 0

Printed in Great Britain by R. & R. Clark, Ltd., Edinburgh

John D. Jones 1972

st published 1972,
Edward Arnold (Publishers) Ltd.,
Maddox Street,
don, W1R 0AN

ds edition ISBN 0 7131 2339 7
r edition ISBN 0 7131 2340 0

eat Britain by R. & R. Clark, Ltd., Edinburgh

Special Topics in Biology Series

Comparative Physiology of Resp

John D. Jones
B.Sc., Ph.D.
Senior Lecturer in Zoology, University of Sheffiel

Fi
by
41
Lo

Boa
Pap

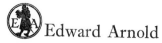 Edward Arnold

Printed in C

Preface

Since its publication in 1941, August Krogh's *Comparative Physiology of Respiratory Mechanisms* has been a great boon to students of respiration. The high esteem in which this book is held is indicated by the great frequency of its citation in textbooks, monographs, reviews and research papers. It gives a concise review of knowledge of respiratory gas exchange (up to 1939) right across the animal kingdom and provides an unrivalled perspective of the field. Generations of undergraduate students have looked to it for guidance and library copies have become increasingly dog-eared since it has unhappily been out of print for many years.

The time seems ripe to attempt another review of this broad subject in a similar spirit of exposition rather than exhaustive compilation, the whole field having taken on a new interest as a result of the brilliant elucidation of the structure of haemoglobin and myoglobin. Recent discoveries in this area have opened up exciting possibilities of interpreting functional characteristics in molecular terms. At the same time there have been very substantial advances in other areas of the subject which well deserve to be brought together. The present account is offered not in any sense to supersede Krogh's classical work but to supplement it, in some senses to broaden it and at the same time to provide a reasonably comprehensive account.

There has been no shortage of excellent review articles and monographs and books covering particular aspects of the subject and, as the text and bibliography will show, I have been happy to draw heavily upon many of these. An attempted perspective view must necessarily take an individual viewpoint and my selection of topics for inclusion is no doubt a highly personal one. I make no apology for what may seem an excessive emphasis on the respiratory pigments (this is an important area and the one I know best) or for discussion of a few topics at very considerable length—to my mind they illustrate particularly well the complexity of the functions and of the relationships with which biology is concerned. Neither do I apologize for what may seem to some readers excessive teleological speculation—frank and self-controlled speculation seems to me to be an essential part of the comparative approach. It is vitally important, however, to keep clearly in mind where facts and adequately substantiated theories end and speculations begin.

In determining the level of approach, the needs of advanced undergraduate students have been principally in mind though it is hoped that their teachers may also find something of value and that workers in this field may be suitably provoked. A fairly thorough documentation of sources has been attempted but reference has frequently been made to textbooks, monographs and reviews rather than to original papers as it was thought this would best serve the interests of overburdened undergraduate readers. At the same time this may help the reader to find his way into many of the areas which I have neglected.

The general form of the book, which owes an obvious debt to Krogh, follows in much expanded form the pattern adopted over a considerable number of years in lecture courses and the detailed methods of presentation of certain topics have evolved in the same context. The range encompassed overall has led far beyond the limits of my personal experience and I am well aware that there will be errors and omissions; I shall be most grateful to any readers who will bring these to my notice.

I am deeply indebted to Professor Drs. H. P. Wolvekamp of the University of Leiden for his thorough reading of the manuscript and for many valuable criticisms and suggestions. Needless to say, for any imperfections which remain I alone am responsible. To numerous other colleagues I am indebted for the patience with which they have allowed me to pick their brains on particular points. Finally, I wish to acknowledge with thanks the energy with which my wife has contributed to the preparation of the manuscript and the patience with which she has supported my efforts.

Sheffield   J. D. J.
1971

Contents

I Introduction

One of the author's more imaginative and perceptive first-year undergraduate students wrote in an examination answer: 'The role of respiratory oxygen is to clear up the debris of the Krebs Cycle'. Indeed, the earth would have been a very different place if the first living organisms had developed the capacity for excreting hydrogen and carbon monoxide.

However, as things are, the utilization of oxygen and the disposal of carbon dioxide are paramount among the functions carried out by all aerobic organisms, the varied aspects of these activities being collectively referred to as respiration. It is customary to divide the field into two distinct parts: internal respiration, the sum of all those enzymatic reactions within the cell by which energy is made available, and external respiration, the mechanisms facilitating the entry of oxygen to and the exit of carbon dioxide from the organism. This work is almost entirely concerned with these exchange mechanisms.

In considering the arrangements for external respiration in the great majority of animals, it is sometimes convenient to distinguish the processes of exchange of the respiratory gases between the body fluids and the environment, from the transport of these gases to and from the tissues where they are chemically engaged. These aspects are, however, closely interrelated and their study constitutes a field of unrivalled interest to the comparative physiologist.

The discipline of comparative physiology owes its existence to the fact that amongst animals, diversity of form and of environmental circumstances have given rise to a multitude of different adaptations subserving the relatively unified patterns of cellular metabolism. Nowhere is this state of affairs better exemplified than in the realm of respiration and it provides the essential justification for asking 'Why?' as well as 'How?'.

Until comparatively recently it was widely held to be scientifically improper to seek for such teleological explanations even in biology. However, many comparative physiologists, undaunted by the shibboleths of orthodoxy, have indulged in teleological speculation and reaped a rich harvest of understanding of the nature of living processes. It is hoped that one of the incidental values of the discussions which follow will be to demonstrate the value of moderate speculation about the functional significance of observed facts in prompting questions capable of experimental investigation. This leads on to a more profound understanding of the facts and of the mechanisms themselves.

Unlike most other exchanges between the animal and its environment, external respiration is essentially a passive process. True, in the interests of efficiency, energy may be expended in moving the medium on one or both sides of the exchange membranes but it is now generally agreed that movement of gas from one medium to another can be fully accounted for on the basis of diffusion alone. Furthermore, with the sole exception of the tracheal systems of insects and some arachnids, we are concerned virtually exclusively with gas diffusion in aqueous solution. It follows that the primary physical factors in the exchange of respiratory gases are the existence of concentration gradients.

These gradients owe their existence fundamentally to the uptake and output activities respectively of the respiring cells but they may be enhanced by the employment of a number of devices in order to minimize the extent which the slowness of diffusion of dissolved gases may limit the activity. An outline of the nature and consequences of these basic physical aspects of respiratory gas exchange is given in the following chapter.

Later we shall see that, with the tendency for animals to become in the course of evolution larger and more active, they make increasing demands for oxygen upon external media which are more or less well suited to supply them. Even if the external supply position is optimal, the exchange across external bounding membranes and subsequent transport to the deeper-lying tissues will often necessitate development of complex morphological and physiological arrangements. The interpretation and understanding of these circulatory and respiratory organ mechanisms is enormously helped by the comparative approach.

Finally the elucidation of the varied roles of respiratory pigments will reveal the crowning subtlety of the whole gas exchange function, the complex integration of all the diverse elements and the great potential for both phylogenetic and ontogenetic adaptation to changes in the external environment and modes of life.

After considering the remarkable diversity and ingenuity of respiratory exchange mechanisms and adaptations, one may pause to wonder why the provision of oxygen to the tissues and concomitant carbon dioxide elimination should be so important. Many highly organized animals can survive and remain in some cases very active when the oxygen supply to the tissues falls far short of their needs. Why then is there evidently such a 'struggle' for oxygen to minimize anaerobic metabolism?

The answer to this question is now familiar, if he thinks about it, to every schoolboy biologist, though even as recently as 25 years ago it might well have eluded the foremost researchers. It is simply that for every gram of food metabolized under fully aerobic conditions in the cell, the potential yield of energy is nearly 20 times greater than would be available under anaerobic conditions. As in human societies, so in the animal kingdom at large there are few who can afford to be really prodigal with their food supplies.

This is a case where in the broadest terms we appear to have a satisfactory answer to the question 'Why?' but to answer in detail the question 'How?' much work still needs to be done. It is hoped that the chapters which follow will suggest to the reader some ways in which our considerable understanding of this field can be further extended.

2 Problems of Diffusion in Respiratory Gas Exchange

Although the proof is of a negative character, it can be asserted with some confidence that respiratory gas exchange rests solely on passive processes of physical diffusion. Early in this century it was held by some physiologists, such as Chr. Bohr and J. S. Haldane, that in man, at least during exercise and after acclimatization to low oxygen pressures, active secretion of oxygen across the pulmonary epithelium could be demonstrated.[73] However, the experimental evidence was not conclusive and indeed many careful comparisons of alveolar and arterial oxygen pressures have put the former at least 1 or 2 mm higher. Krogh and others[128,129] have calculated that the experimentally determined rates of diffusion of oxygen in living tissues and the shortness of the limiting diffusion pathways are sufficient to account for the highest observed rates of oxygen uptake. For reasons which are discussed below, the potential flux of carbon dioxide is some 25 times greater than that of oxygen, so there is even less need to postulate secretion in this case. The gas gland of the teleost swimbladder (possibly also the hydrostatic organs of some invertebrates) and the choroid rete of the teleost eye are the only tissues in which active movement of oxygen against a concentration gradient has been clearly established.

It follows that some appreciation of the factors bearing on the rate of diffusion of oxygen (and of carbon dioxide) is fundamental to the discussion of mechanisms of external respiration. In all cases, with the exception of insect tracheal systems, we are concerned with diffusion of gases in solution, so we may start with the question of solubility.

Solubility of gases

The amount of a gas which is dissolved in water in equilibrium with a gaseous phase depends on α, the absorption (or Bunsen) coefficient. This is defined as the volume of dry gas (measured at S.T.P.) taken up by one volume of water from an atmosphere in which the pressure of the said gas is 760 mm. The quantity of any gas absorbed is thus proportional to the pressure of that gas and independent of any other gases which may be present in the gaseous or aqueous phases. The concentration of a dissolved gas may therefore be expressed either in terms of its actual amount (by volume or weight) per unit volume of solution or of partial pressure* (measured in mm of Hg or torr). Given the absorption coefficient the alternative expressions are readily interconvertible. In contexts involving the activity of the gas, partial pressure is the appropriate form and in the case of dissolved gas this is commonly referred to (by physiologists at least) as the gas tension.*

* In either case abbreviated to pO_2, pCO_2 etc.

By definition, the partial tension of a dissolved gas is equal to its partial pressure in the gas phase with which it is in equilibrium.

The solubility of gases is diminished by two biologically important variables, namely increases in temperature and in concentration of dissolved solids. The extent of the influence of these factors is illustrated in Table 2.1. A numerical

Table 2.1 Absorption coefficients for carbon dioxide, nitrogen and oxygen in water at various temperatures and for oxygen at various salinities. 20‰ Cl⁻ corresponds to normal sea-water.

°C	CO_2	N_2	0‰Cl	O_2 10‰Cl	20‰Cl
0	1.713	0.0239	0.0489	0.0434	0.0379
10	1.194	0.0196	0.0380	0.0341	0.0301
20	0.878	0.0164	0.0310	0.0281	0.0251
30	0.665	0.0138	0.0261	0.0235	0.0209

example will clarify the above considerations. Thus a body of pure water in contact with the normal atmosphere will come to equilibrium in a manner which is precisely calculable. If the barometric pressure is 760 mm and the temperature 20°C, the gas mixture at the water surface will have the following composition: water vapour 17.5 mm; nitrogen 78.08% of 760 – 17.5 = 580 mm; oxygen 20.95% of 760 – 17.5 = 155.5 mm; carbon dioxide 0.03% of 760 – 17.5 = 0.22 mm. At 20°C the absorption coefficients are for oxygen 0.0310; for nitrogen 0.0164 and for carbon dioxide 0.878. Hence, the concentrations of dissolved gases in ml/l are:

$$O_2 \quad 0.0310 \times 1000 \times 155.5/760 = 6.34 \text{ (or } pO_2 = 155.5 \text{ mm)}$$
$$N_2 \quad 0.0164 \times 1000 \times 580/760 = 12.5 \text{ (or } pN_2 = 580.0 \text{ mm)}$$
$$CO_2 \quad 0.878 \times 1000 \times 0.22/760 = 0.25 \text{ (or } pCO_2 = 0.22 \text{ mm)}$$

Diffusion of gases in solution

The strict treatment of diffusion of gases in solution according to kinetic theory is complex and need not be attempted here, but certain basic principles which have been determined empirically should be stated. The rates of diffusion of different gases in the same solvent are directly proportional to their respective absorption coefficients and inversely proportional to the square roots of their molecular weights. The net effect of change in temperature, which alters the absorption coefficient on the one hand and the internal friction of the solvent on the other, is to increase or decrease the diffusion rate in water about 1% for every degree by which the temperature is higher or lower than 20°C. The salinity of the medium affects diffusion rate by virtue of its effect on the absorption coefficient.

We may therefore express the rate of diffusion of a particular gas in absolute terms by reference to its diffusion coefficient at a particular temperature. This coefficient is usually defined as the volume in ml of gas diffusing in 1 minute along a pathway which is 1 cm² in area and 1 cm in length when the partial pressure difference between the ends is 760 mm. This coefficient serves equally well for diffusion in the gaseous or aqueous phases but it is important to realize that in either case the concentration (or more exactly the activity) gradient is measured in partial pressure of gas, not, as might be expected in the case of dissolved gases, in ml or mg per litre.

This latter proviso is important when considering the movement of a gas between two media in which its solubility is different. For example, in marine teleosts the total salt content of the blood is only about one-third that of the external medium, so that if both blood and sea-water were in equilibrium with the atmosphere the concentration of all dissolved gases would be higher in the blood than in the sea-water, although by definition the partial tension of each gas would be the same in both media and no diffusion exchange would occur. Conversely diffusion exchange would occur across the gill epithelium when the dissolved gas concentrations are equal; indeed up to a point inward diffusion can occur against a 'concentration' gradient. This apparent anomaly (which arises from the erroneous equating of concentration with activity of dissolved gases) will be reversed in the case of hyperosmotic freshwater animals.

The experimental determination of diffusion coefficients of dissolved gases is a difficult operation and the values obtained by Krogh in 1919 for diffusion in some animal tissues are still the best we have. His figures for oxygen are given in Table 2.2. The relative diffusion rates of different gases in solution in the same fluid are governed by the net effect of variation in absorption coefficient and molecular weight (see above) and the relationships are temperature dependent. At 20°C the carbon dioxide flux* is about 26 times greater than that of oxygen.

Table 2.2 Diffusion coefficients of oxygen at 20°C. Volume in ml/(min × cm² × cm × atm). These data are sometimes given as diffusion *constants* for a path length of 1 μm in which case the figures are 10^4 times greater. (Krogh[124])

In air	11.0
water	0.000034
gelatine 20% solution	0.000028
muscle	0.000014
connective tissue	0.0000115
chitin	0.0000013†
india rubber	0.0000077

† Later misquoted by Krogh[128] and by other authors subsequently.

* It is important to distinguish between the amount of gas moving over a given distance in unit time (flux) and the velocity of individual molecules.

Limitations of diffusion

Krogh was probably the first to attempt to express in quantitative terms the implications of the slowness of dissolved gas diffusion for the supply of oxygen to respiring tissues. He showed (see his monograph of 1941[128]) that for a homogeneous spherical organism of radius 1 cm with a respiration rate constant throughout its depth at 100 ml O_2/kg/hr, the limiting external pressure of oxygen for gas to reach the centre would be about 25 atmospheres relying on diffusion alone. Theoretically, the limiting pressure difference should be proportional to the square of the radius but since metabolic rate is usually found to be proportional not to weight (or r^3) but more nearly to $W^{2/3}$ or surface area (r^2) (see p. 24), the difference will be more closely dependent on the simple radius (see footnote p. 7).

As a rough generalization Krogh concluded that when metabolism is fairly high, diffusion alone can provide sufficient oxygen from a normal atmosphere for animals of up to 1 mm diameter only. Even this figure is based on the assumption that there is adequate external convection to prevent any gradient occurring outside the animal. On the other hand, a sphere represents the most adverse surface/volume ratio in this context and any deviation from the spherical will improve conditions for diffusion. Threadlike forms such as the larger nematodes constitute an obvious illustration of this point. Sponges constitute a different kind of exception with their continuous circulation of well-aerated water through a structure having a surface area which is practically proportional to the mass; in this case oxygen supply is virtually independent of size. Another group capable of maintaining large size on the basis of diffusion exchange alone are the coelenterates. The explanation in this case is based on two unusual factors: the very low percentage of metabolically active tissue and the attenuated nature of the active ectodermal and endodermal layers.

Diffusion with circulation

The first development required to facilitate increase in size along with a high metabolic rate is an internal convection system or circulation. If it is assumed that the diffusion processes are limited to the layer ('cuticle') separating the external medium from the internal circulating medium, the limiting external pO_2 for the maintenance of uptake at 100 ml/kg/hr by a spherical organism of 1 cm radius and 50 μm cuticle thickness is about one-quarter of an atmosphere. In practice an allowance must also be made for a further diffusion from the circulation into the respiring tissues and for some lack of complete equilibration between the internal and external media across the cuticle. Adequate circulation rate is also essential.

If metabolism were proportional to weight, the limiting pressure difference would be proportional to the radius of the sphere and a size limitation would be imposed. When, however, metabolism is proportional to $W^{2/3}$ or surface area this limitation theoretically disappears,* though in practice other factors become limiting (see below). Respiratory gas exchange through the general body surface in association with a circulatory system is found in leeches, some polychaete and all oligochaete annelids. Indeed, in the latter group this type of provision serves for animals weighing up to about 1 kg (e.g. tropical earthworms such as *Rhinodrilus fafner*, which may reach a length of 2.1 m and a diameter of 24 mm and *Megascolides australis* which reaches a length of 2.2 m).[205]

A number of factors ultimately render an unspecialized body surface inadequate for gas exchange but the limiting size cannot be defined in general terms, depending as it does on a multitude of aspects of the animal's habitat, mode of life, bodily organization etc. In respect of carbon dioxide elimination, these factors are much less critical than they are for oxygen and in amphibia, for example, cutaneous exchange of carbon dioxide predominates over pulmonary exchange at all times, particularly during the non-breeding seasons (p. 44). The limitation rests on the provision of an adequate area of surface separated from the blood by a sufficiently thin diffusion barrier to permit an adequate flux of oxygen. Area is limited by the total surface of the animal and the effective thinness is limited by considerations of mechanical protection and the need to limit flux of water due to osmotic gradient or dessication.

Circulation with respiratory organs

Sooner or later the demand for oxygen will overtake the limitations of the above mentioned factors and further advance in size or activity will depend on the development of specialized respiratory organs. These are customarily called 'gills' when they take the form of evaginations from the surface, as in most aquatic forms, and 'lungs' when they are invaginations from the surface, as in most terrestrial (or physiologically more aptly, 'aerial') forms. In either case it becomes possible for the blood to be brought into much more intimate contact with the external medium and for the latter to be renewed at the respiratory epithelium in an efficient manner (p. 47).

It must be strongly emphasized that the limitations of the general surface diffusion condition can in no way be improved by the development of respiratory

---

* For diffusion exchange alone the formula employed is $C_0 = \dfrac{Ar^2}{6D}$, where C_0 is pO_2 at surface in atmospheres, A is O_2 consumption in ml/g/min, r is radius in cm, D is diffusion coefficient in ml/atm × cm × cm². That is to say $C_0 \propto Ar^2$; but if O_2 uptake is in reality proportional to surface area (r^2) rather than weight (r^3) then $C_0 \propto \dfrac{A}{r^3} \times r^2 \times r^2 = Ar$. For trans-cuticular diffusion plus circulation the formula is $C_0 = \dfrac{ArT}{3D}$, where T is thickness of cuticle. That is to say $C_0 \propto Ar$ which (if $A \propto W^{2/3}$) becomes $C_0 \propto A \times \dfrac{r^2}{r^3} \times r = A$. i.e. limiting pressure is independent of size. In practice $A \propto W^{0.75}$ or thereabouts not to $W^{2/3}$ (p. 24); some size dependent limitation therefore remains.

organs without a circulatory system which supplies the organs and the rest of the body. Because of the limiting rate of diffusion within the tissues, a respiratory organ can only absorb more oxygen (and eliminate more carbon dioxide) than is required for its own metabolism if some internal convection exists to pass on the benefits of improved exchange with the medium. The designation of certain appendages (such as the so called 'blood gills' of culicine and chironomid larvae) as gills is therefore quite invalid.

Circulation with respiratory pigments

Another factor limiting the development of high rates of gas exchange is the rate at which the blood, charged with oxygen and carbon dioxide, can be circulated between the tissues and the respiratory epithelium. This limit may (as in the case of the oligochaetes) be reached even before the need for special respiratory organs becomes apparent. Given that, for hydrodynamic and other reasons, there is a definite upper limit to circulation rate, then a point will be reached at which the demand for oxygen will exceed the capacity of the blood to carry it in solution. At this stage in the evolution of a group it is appropriate (and apparently not very difficult) to develop a specific respiratory carrier for oxygen, thus increasing the oxygen capacity of the blood. A fuller discussion of the physical factors additionally involved in this case will be deferred to Chapter 9.

Generalized respiratory system

At this point it may be useful to summarize the main characteristics of a general-ized system in an animal in possession of both circulation and respiratory organs. This is attempted in Fig. 2.1. The central rectangle drawn as a continuous double line represents the circulating blood, in contact at the left, with the respiratory epithelium and at the right, with the tissues. Oxygen diffuses from left to right (and carbon dioxide from right to left) at both these barriers. The varying heights of the dotted lines represent, in a purely qualitative way, the partial pressures of oxygen in the blood and in the various tissues. The blood vessel walls are repre-sented in thickness only in the capillaries, where significant gas exchange occurs. The respiratory epithelium may be seen as a window on to the external world and in the case illustrated it takes the form of a gill with the external medium running counter-current to the blood. This arrangement which is anatomically well developed in the most efficient gill-breathers, the teleosts, ensures that the external medium comes as close to equilibrium with the blood as possible and at the maximum pO_2 (p. 49).

In the case of lung-breathers with efficient ventilation, the pulmonary (alveolar) pO_2 remains virtually constant and the dotted pO_2 gradient lines across the re-spiratory epithelium would converge on the point p_e (alveolar pO_2). Oxygen available in the external medium at tension p_e is thus finally delivered to the centre of a tissue cell most remote from the distal end of a capillary at tension p_c; a cell similarly remote from the proximal end of a capillary would receive

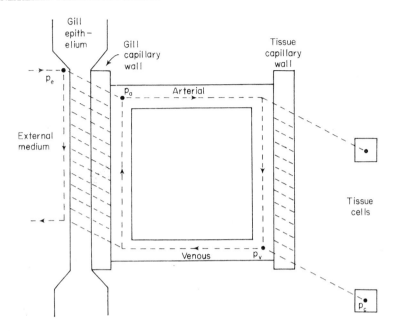

Fig. 2.1 Schematic representation of a generalized system for oxygen exchange with circulation and a respiratory organ. The broken lines represent not only the movement of the gas by convection or diffusion but also (in a qualitative way) the partial pressure relationships in the external medium, vascular system and tissues and the intervening diffusion gradients. (For explanation see text)

oxygen at a correspondingly higher tension. p_a and p_v represent the pO_2 of arterial and venous blood respectively.

The relationship of the various pO_2 points will depend firstly on the diffusion characteristics of the two diffusion barriers (diffusion coefficient and thickness). Secondly, the rate of flow through the two capillary beds may be significant, especially in the respiratory organ, in influencing the extent of equilibration of the blood with the external medium. A sluggish flow will facilitate a more complete equilibration but may yet (if the extent of the capillary is not optimal in relation to the total circulation rate) diminish the net transport rate of oxygen by the overall circulation. Thirdly, the steepness of the final diffusion gradient will be governed by the diffusion characteristics of the tissue in relation to its metabolic rate. The higher the oxygen consumption of the cells (given a constant capillary supply) the lower will p_c become. Finally, the overall pressure drop in delivering a given amount of oxygen to the ultimate destination will be governed by the relationship between the oxygen content of the blood and its pO_2; the more oxygen can be taken up or given up by the blood for a given change in pO_2 the better. This aspect will be more fully explored in Chapter 9.

Final diffusion pathway

Clearly, to sustain a high level of aerobic metabolism within the limits of a reasonable circulation rate, many factors must combine to ensure that p_v is high enough to satisfy this simple equation:

$$Q_{O_2} = K\,(p_v - p_c)$$

The oxygen consumption (Q_{O_2}) is limited to the rate at which oxygen moves from the capillary blood to the respiring cell and this is governed by the difference in pO_2 between the ends of this diffusion path and the diffusion characteristics (including path length) of the tissue between (K). In defining the upper end of the tissue gradient in terms of venous tension (p_v) we are putting the matter in the worst possible light; for cells deriving their oxygen from the proximal end of the capillary, the appropriate tension is p_a. However, in the discussion which follows we are really most interested in the limiting case.

Rather little is known about the diffusion coefficients of oxygen in living tissues beyond the few values given in Table 2.2. Krogh was the first to attempt determinations of the length of the final diffusion path in order to calculate the limiting value of p_v–p_c necessary to ensure the satisfaction of known metabolic rates. His observations were confined to vertebrate muscular tissues in which the capillaries are arranged in a rather regular and parallel fashion. This was the first work to demonstrate that in addition to the tendency for individual capillaries to dilate in working muscles, the number of open capillaries increases with the demand for oxygen so that increased Q_{O_2} is at least in part met by a shortening of the diffusion path and so increasing K. Thus in guinea pig skeletal muscle the number of open capillaries (determined by histological methods) in a cross section of 1 mm² increased from 30 at rest to 3000 when working maximally, with a consequent reduction of maximum diffusion distance from 100 to 10 μm. The corresponding reduction in the limiting value of p_v–p_c was calculated to be from 45 to 1.2 mm. In the frog there was a similar, though less dramatic, change in limiting pO_2 gradient from 10 mm at rest to 1.2 mm in the working muscle, the number of open capillaries having increased from 10 to 325 per mm² and the maximum diffusion path having decreased from 180 to 30 μm.[125]

In this, as in so many other aspects of respiratory physiology, Krogh's pioneering efforts have not been superseded.* The determination of diffusion path lengths in tissues is the most critical factor in calculation of the dynamics of oxygen exchange between blood and tissues and in spite of subsequent use of more sophisticated methods, Krogh's values are as certain as any later ones. It is of considerable interest to compare his calculated conclusions with those more recently obtained, by more or less direct experimental approaches to the same problem.

Experimentally one must attempt to determine separately, limiting values for intracellular pO_2 (p_c) and venous pO_2 (p_v). Direct absolute measurements

---

* A fine summary of his work on capillaries was published in 1929 and reprinted in 1959 with a posthumous biographical essay.[127]

of p_c are at present virtually impossible, even with the advent of micro-oxygen electrodes (because of calibration difficulties). Indirectly, it is possible to determine the critical pO_2 below which the Q_{O_2} of an *in vitro* mitochondrial suspension begins to fall or to measure *in vivo*, by fluorimetry, the onset of reduction of the pyridene nucleotides (NAD and FAD) as a function of pO_2.[29] Both these techniques indicate that the limiting value of p_c for fully aerobic metabolism is about 1 mm or less. Limiting values of p_V have been determined by monitoring flow rate, p_a and p_V for a single muscle (the gastrocnemius) *in situ*, in a dog which was made progressively hypoxic by rebreathing. In the resting muscle oxygen consumption remained constant at 5 $\mu l/g/min$ until p_a and p_V dropped to 50 mm and 30 mm respectively; when the muscle was stimulated its Q_{O_2} rose to 40 $\mu l/g/min$ and remained steady until p_a and p_V dropped to 35 and 10 mm respectively.[162] Thus, we arrive at limiting values for p_V–p_c, in the dog gastrocnemius, of 29 mm at rest and 9 mm at work. It is unlikely that the eightfold increase in oxygen consumption of the intact muscle represents maximal work and there was evidence that the capillary bed was not fully open. These figures may be compared with Krogh's calculated gradients of 45 mm at rest and 1.2 mm for maximum work in guinea pig muscle.

It would be extremely interesting to compare experimental and calculated limiting gradients for the same muscle; this might help to establish whether or not diffusion facilitation by myoglobin in mammalian muscle cells is a significant factor in intramuscular diffusion (see p. 135).

As we shall see later (p. 23) there is a striking inverse correlation between metabolic rate and body weight. It is interesting, therefore, to find that small mammals (bat and mouse) are assisted in the maintenance of their relatively high metabolic rate by having a greater density of capillaries and hence shorter final diffusion pathways than larger mammals. This inverse correlation of capillary density with body weight does not hold throughout the range of sizes investigated (bat to cow).[169]

Adequacy of final diffusion

The following conclusions seem to be justified at the present time: resting mammalian muscles will receive oxygen at an adequate rate and pressure provided that the circulatory provision does not cause the venous pO_2 to fall below about 45 to 30 mm; in working muscles, thanks to the opening-up of the capillary bed, venous pO_2 may drop to much lower levels (in the range of 10 to 1 mm) before aerobic metabolism is impaired. This does not preclude the possibility of momentary deficiency in a muscle going suddenly into strong contraction, pending the opening-up of additional capillaries; in this situation myoglobin is thought to act as a short-term oxygen store (see p. 135). It might appear that the smaller limiting gradient required by the working muscle indicates an over-compensation by the capillary bed adjustment but, of course, it is precisely by a lowering of the limiting venous tension that the necessary increase in blood oxygen turnover is achieved, so ensuring delivery of the increased volume of the gas without excessive increase in circulation rate.

In trying to establish the potential adequacy of diffusion to move oxygen from the capillaries to the cells we have overlooked one possibly significant additional factor; this is the circulation of intercellular fluid. Little attention has been paid to this as a means of oxygen transport but the slowness of the flow precludes it as a dramatic factor.

Our knowledge of the circumstances at the capillary/cellular level* in vertebrates is scanty but for invertebrates it is practically non-existent. In those forms with vascular systems, tissues are generally less well furnished with capillaries than those of higher vertebrates. Accordingly, lower limits of venous pO_2 may be more critical, even though metabolic rates are generally lower. This is no doubt offset in part by a greater tolerance of anaerobiosis in many forms but the properties of respiratory pigments may also be involved. These are questions to which we shall return in later chapters.

* For fuller discussion of this question see Forster[54] and Longmuir.[144]

3 The Respiratory Medium—
Aerial *v.* Aquatic

The question is sometimes asked: 'Is aerial respiration more efficient than aquatic respiration?' Essentially, attempts to answer such questions are fraught with danger because final conclusions tend to depend on anthropomorphic notions of success. However, a comparison of aerial and aquatic respiration can be a useful exercise if it illuminates the nature of the problems involved.

Oxygen in air and water

As respiratory media, air and water exhibit a number of striking differences of which the most important are oxygen content, density and viscosity.

One litre of dry air contains 209.5 ml of oxygen, equivalent at STP to $0.2095/22.4$ or 0.935×10^{-2} moles. A similar volume of water in equilibrium with the atmosphere contains a much smaller quantity of dissolved oxygen depending on temperature, barometric pressure and the concentration of dissolved solids (see Table 2.1). For distilled water and sea-water at 20°C and normal barometric pressure the volumes are 6.34 ml and 5.11 ml respectively. Air saturated water is not in equilibrium with dry air but with air at 100% R.H. hence $pO_2 = 20.95\%$ of 760–v.p. (see p. 4).

In spite of the great difference in oxygen content of air and water the pO_2 is almost the same. Thus, provided that the uptake of oxygen by the respiratory organ is not allowed to cause a local oxygen depletion and that internal conditions are the same, the gradient across the respiratory epithelium and hence the rate of diffusion will be the same in either medium. The first qualification is ideal but can come close to fulfilment in an animal with an efficient system of ventilation.*

Irrigation and ventilation

In aquatic animals irrigation depends on some mechanical means of moving a stream of water over the gills. Arrangements range from the lateral cilia on the gill lamellae of bivalve molluscs, amphioxus and ascidians to the branchial pump of fishes. Tubicolous polychaetes depend on ciliary currents (*Nephtys*, the spionids) or peristaltic (*Arenicola*) or undulating (*Chaetopterus*) movements of the body wall for irrigation of the burrow. Crustacea commonly depend on undulating (vibrating) appendages. In all cases where irrigation is efficient and

---

* Contrary to the practice of many writers, we shall reserve the term 'ventilation' for respiratory movement of air and use the term 'irrigation' for movement of water over the respiratory surfaces.

air-saturated water is available, the pO_2 on the outside of the respiratory epithelium will not fall far short of the atmospheric level. Production of a water stream specifically for gill irrigation may be absent in animals living in flowing water or swimming continuously.

The supposed advantage of gills in not having a stagnant layer of water outside the gas exchange epithelium may be illusory. In a recent mathematical analysis of oxygen transfer in the fish gill it was concluded that because the flow over the secondary lamellae is normally laminar, there is a stationary layer which may contribute 80–90% of the total diffusion resistance.[87]

In lung-breathing terrestrial animals the situation is otherwise. Only vertebrates have developed ventilation lungs in which the gas content can be actively renewed. Even then there is a marked alveolar oxygen deficiency which cannot be eliminated because of the tidal nature of the renewal mechanism. This is in marked contrast to the through-flow arrangement which characterizes all the more efficient gill irrigation mechanisms.

In man the resting volume of the lung at expiration is about 2.9 l. Inspiration introduces about 0.5 l of atmospheric air, of which about 0.36 l reaches the alveoli, the remainder filling the dead space of the trachea, bronchi and bronchioles. Consequently, fresh atmospheric air is always diluted by a much larger volume of oxygen-deficient residual air and the alveolar pO_2 does not exceed 105 mm. This situation is not significantly affected by the larger proportion of tidal air during exercise, because the regulatory mechanisms which govern gas exchange through ventilation are geared to maintain the constancy of alveolar gas composition.

The situation is essentially the same in other lung-breathing vertebrates, although it is possible that birds can exploit the ambient pO_2 to a somewhat greater extent than mammals by virtue of the much more elaborate architecture of the lung and associated structures. There is as yet no agreed description of the detailed air flow through the air-sacs, mesobronchi, lateral and parabronchi[88] but it seems that in spite of the overall tidal pattern, there is a through-flow in close proximity to the gas exchange surfaces (air capillaries of the parabronchi). This probably results in a higher 'alveolar' pO_2 than is obtainable with a simple tidal pattern; in the abdominal air sacs 17–19% oxygen is found, compared with 14–15% in the alveoli in man. At the same time arterial pO_2 reaches 114 mm in the pigeon with a corresponding decrease in the oxygen affinity of the haemoglobin.[207]

In air-breathing invertebrates lung-like structures lack deliberate ventilation mechanisms, maintenance of pulmonary pO_2 depending on diffusion alone. The lung books of arachnids communicate with the exterior by spiracles which remain permanently open and a fairly constant pulmonary pO_2 results. In pulmonate gastropods, on the other hand, the pulmonary aperture in the mantle is only opened periodically so that a cycle of pulmonary pO_2 results. When this periodic opening is restricted by diving behaviour in aquatic forms very extensive changes occur and make their impact on the whole pattern of external respiration (p. 116). Thus in *Planorbis corneus* and *Lymnaea stagnalis* the pO_2 rises to 120–135 mm before closure (higher than the alveolar level of mammals despite the lack of active ventilation) and may fall as low as 20 mm before re-opening.[106] In some insects muscular action serves to ventilate at least the main longitudinal tracheal trunks but movement along the major part of the system is passive. The question of irrigation/ventilation arrangements is more fully discussed in Chapter 7.

Utilization

Although maintenance of the highest possible pO_2 at the respiratory epithelium is in principle desirable it is clearly not always possible or economic; in any case other factors, operative inside the epithelium, also govern the rate of diffusion at this barrier. An important concept relating external and internal factors is that of utilization, which in the present context we define as the percentage withdrawal of oxygen from the respiratory medium. [In mammalian respiration this term is sometimes used to designate the difference in oxygen content between arterial and venous blood.] Utilization is determined by comparing the oxygen content of the inhalent and exhalent respiratory currents and the concept is only of use when these can be distinguished.

Amongst groups of aquatic animals (where utilization is measurable) we can distinguish two classes. In fishes and in cephalopods utilization normally exceeds 50% and may reach 80%; in polychaetes 30–70% and in crustacea 43–76% utilization values are found.[16] In sponges (6–40%), lamellibranchs (3–10%) ascidians (4–7%) the values are almost always much lower.[16] Similar values have been found in an extensive investigation by Hazelhoff.[78] It is suggested that the low level of utilization in the second class reflects the dependence on a higher irrigation rate of the concomitant function of filter feeding rather than of gas exchange.

The very high utilization in fishes is undoubtedly favoured by the counter-current flow of water and blood on opposing sides of the respiratory epithelium (Fig. 7.4). As a result of this arrangement there is a potential equilibrium of efferent blood with inhalent water, which is clearly more favourable than between efferent blood and exhalent water. Parallel flow exchange can approach the efficiency of counter-current exchange if the contributory medium flows faster (and in greater quantity) than the uptake medium but in this case the utilization would be low and the work involved in irrigation excessive. The importance of counter-current flow in fish respiration may be judged by the fact that if the flow over the gill lamellae is experimentally reversed in the tench, utilization drops to below 10%.[89]

The advantageous employment of the counter-current principle has been presumed in a number of invertebrate groups but experimental verification is scanty. Yonge[236] has claimed that blood flow through the gill filaments in the opposite direction to the flow of water outside is a constant feature of the Mollusca. However, his figure and description of the arrangements in the cuttle fish *Sepia* indicate that the main water flow does not conform to this principle.

Since it is precisely in the cephalopods, with their very high levels of utilization, that counter-current flow would be expected, an experimental study in this group would be most valuable. In the shore crab *Carcinus maenas*, the presence of counter-current flow is now firmly established by the experimental study of Hughes et al,[91] but utilization proves to be low (7–23%). Existence of dead spaces in the branchial cavity and wide separation of the gill lamellae, low permeability of lamella membranes and inadequate perfusion of lamella capillaries were suggested factors limiting oxygen uptake from the water stream. The gill area relative to body weight is quite equal to that of many active fishes.

Utilization in the lungs of higher vertebrates is intermediate between the extremes found in aquatic animals. In man the crude comparison between inspired air (20.9% O_2) and expired air (16.4%) gives a value of about 22%,* while in the pigeon it is somewhat higher (20.9% v. 14.5%) at 31%.[207]

Cost of ventilation and irrigation

The question of respiratory regulation is discussed in Chapter 11 but one aspect of this question, which bears on the comparison of air and water as respiratory media, should be mentioned here. In the face of a drop in the ambient pO_2 or a rise in the demand for oxygen, some animals, especially those whose normal utilization is not very high, can increase the level while irrigation rate remains more or less unchanged (p. 19). However, those normally with high utilization generally have to rely on increased irrigation to meet respiratory stress. For aquatic animals this may have serious consequences because of the relatively high cost of irrigation. Water is about 1800 times more dense and about 100 times more viscous than air, not to mention about 25 to 30 times less rich in oxygen content.

In the eel a drop in oxygen concentration from air saturation to 4 ml/l is accompanied by a 40% increase in oxygen uptake; practically the whole of this rise is accounted for by the greater activity of the branchial muscles in producing a five-fold increase in irrigation rate. At this higher level the cost represents about 30% of the total metabolism; there is no significant alteration in utilization. In man, on the other hand, with an equally fixed utilization, the cost of ventilation at 5 times the resting level amounts to only about 5% of the total metabolism.

The cost of irrigation has a special significance for aquatic animals in relation to temperature change, as Hughes[89] has pointed out. The resting metabolism of the goldfish increases some 28 times (observed O_2 uptake) when the temperature is raised from 5 to 35°C; at the same time the oxygen content of air-saturated water falls from 9 to 5 ml/l. In consequence, even if the utilization could be held constant over this range (which is doubtful), the irrigation would need to be increased by a factor of 46. A very interesting discussion of various quantitative aspects of external respiration in fishes has been given by Alexander.[3]

* Account should be taken of somewhat variable differences in RH and volume of inspired and expired air—volume difference is due to RQ less than 1.

Respiratory organs and water loss

A final contrast between aerial and aquatic respiration takes us into the realm of water relations. Membranes adapted to the exchange of respiratory gases inevitably permit the movement of other readily diffusible molecules. The osmotic flux of water (and to a lesser extent of salts) can be countered by appropriate and well-tried physiological measures—active exchange of salts with the medium and renal regulation—but evaporative loss of water from the moist skin or from the lung due to difference in R.H. between inspired and expired air, may in extreme environments only be countered by extreme behavioural adaptations. The nocturnal and fossorial habits of small desert mammals, reptiles and amphibia illustrate the point. In this connection it is interesting to recall that in reliance upon fat for energy production, the fasting camel experiences a substantial increase in metabolic water production. This is, however, more than offset by the additional evaporative water loss associated with the uptake of the greater volume of oxygen required to metabolize this substrate.[195]

It has only recently been appreciated how much this evaporative loss is reduced in small mammals and in birds by a kind of counter-current heat exchange mechanism in the respiratory passages. Inspired air is warmed and humidified on its passage through the upper respiratory tract and the walls of the passages are correspondingly cooled. Expired air, which is initially saturated with water vapour at body temperature, is cooled during its return passage and some of its water recondensed.[196]

Returning to the question with which we started this chapter—a categorical answer is clearly out of the question. The respiratory exchange mechanisms of the most active gill-breathers—fishes and cephalopods—are remarkably efficient by any standards, up to the point where the law of diminishing returns overthrows the irrigation mechanism. On the other hand, the high demands of warm-blooded life have never been satisfied except by air-breathing.

4 Availability of Oxygen

Before embarking on a detailed consideration of the nature of respiratory adaptations, it is desirable to review briefly and in general terms the physical availability of oxygen in different habitats. For the moment it will be sufficient to note the gross physical characteristics of the environment or micro-habitat, though, as we shall see in later chapters, an animal's behaviour patterns may significantly influence these characteristics; this is especially true of tubicolous animals.

The atmosphere

The supply of oxygen for aerobic metabolism is ultimately, if not immediately, governed by the nature of the earth's atmosphere. This is (in the dry state) a remarkably constant mixture of 20.95% oxygen, 0.03% carbon dioxide, 78.0% nitrogen and 1.0% argon and other rare gases. The addition of a variable amount of water vapour does not alter the relationship of the other components to each other, though it does lower the absolute content of a given volume of air and, perhaps more important, the partial pressures of the other components. At sea-level when the barometer stands at 760 mm, pO_2 in dry air would be 159.2 mm, while at 20°C (v.p. of water 17.5 mm) and 50% R.H. the figure would be reduced to 20.95 (760–17.5 × 0.5) i.e. 157.4 mm.

With increasing altitude barometric pressure decreases, though the proportions of the mixture remain virtually unchanged and by 5000 m the pO_2 is down to 88 mm. As we saw in the previous chapter, ventilation in lung-breathers is relatively not a costly process so the fall in oxygen concentration at high altitude is of comparatively little consequence but the much diminished available pO_2 at the outer side of the respiratory epithelium is of profound significance, especially for warm-blooded species. Respiratory adaptation to high altitude is discussed in Chapter 11.

Terrestrial habitats

Because of the high rate of diffusion of gases terrestrial micro-habitats are not normally liable to oxygen depletion but one kind of essentially aerial environment is characterized by serious variations of pO_2. In the soil of fields and woodlands pO_2s very close to atmospheric are found even at depths of 30 cm but heavy rain may seal the interstices at the surface preventing free diffusion exchange. In this case, due to the activities of soil organisms, the pO_2 can fall rapidly to very low levels with corresponding rise in pCO_2 and it may be several days before optimal conditions are restored.

Aquatic habitats

The availability of oxygen in aquatic environments is subject to many complex influences and limitations of oxygen supply are more often encountered. Although, given a sufficient rate of irrigation, air-saturated fresh water and sea-water are media potentially as satisfactory as air (see previous chapter), the progressive reduction of oxygen solubility with rise in salinity and temperature may tax the irrigation capacity of an animal and make the prevention of a drastic drop in pO_2 at the respiratory surface impossible. The effect of temperature on irrigation in the goldfish has already been mentioned (p. 16); such a position is aggravated at high salinities. Apparently, in response to this situation there is a direct correlation between haemoglobin concentration and salinity in the brine shrimp *Artemia salina* taken from salt pans in which salinity ranges from 120 to $280^0/_{00}$.[69]

For free-living marine animals the problem of a substantial drop in ambient pO_2 below air-saturation seldom arises. Convection due to wind and temperature gradients ensures a very thorough mixing down to great depths. Oxygen originating from the atmosphere and from photosynthetic activities in the surface layers will generally be well distributed, though there are a few exceptions, such as localities in the Black Sea and in the Gulf of Panama where conditions for adequate circulation are absent.

Adequate mixing also ensures high oxygen levels in rivers unless they are very slow flowing with high organic content as is often the case in the tropics; in recent times industrial and sewage pollution have also become serious factors governing oxygen availability in many rivers. Seasonal circulatory breakdown often occurs in lakes with depths of about 10 m or more due to the occurrence of the thermocline. Below this level very serious oxygen depletion may occur as a result of oxidative activities of bottom organisms but oxygen levels remain high above the thermocline. In ditches and ponds conditions are very variable depending on the balance between equilibration at the surface, photosynthetic activities and oxidative activities. High concentrations of organic debris encouraging bacterial oxidations may render not only the bottom deposits and adjacent water layer anaerobic but also cause a marked depletion in the upper layers. The fluctuation between photosynthetic and oxidative activities of submerged plants can produce quite remarkable diurnal cycles. In warm sunny weather the shallow ditches of the Dutch polderlands may exhibit a diurnal pO_2 swing from 10 to 500 mm[106] (see Fig. 4.1).

Apart from organically rich bottom deposits there are few truly anaerobic aquatic habitats. One of these is found in tropical swamps e.g. the papyrus swamps of East Africa. Here the temperature so favours the bacterial breakdown of dead plant material that the water is completely devoid of oxygen to within 1 mm or so of the surface.[27,109] In spite of this a number of gastropods and oligochaetes have been able to adapt themselves to the pursuit of a reasonably aerobic existence.[14]

Finally, reference must be made to the supposedly oxygen-free conditions which are a feature of the habitat of many intestinal parasites. Here none of the

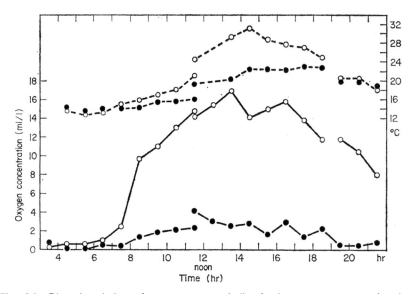

Fig. 4.1 Diurnal variation of temperature and dissolved oxygen concentration in a shallow drainage ditch (15 cm deep) in the Dutch polderlands. Records of two consecutive sunny days in June. o---o surface and ●---● bottom temperature; o——o surface and ●——● bottom oxygen concentration. This ditch, the habitat of the gastropods *Planorbis* and *Lymnaea* discussed on p. 116 et seq., was choked with aquatic plants. The high rate of photosynthesis together with lack of convection resulted in dissolved oxygen concentration rising to a maximum of 17 ml/l near the surface; with a temperature of 30°C this corresponds to a pO_2 of 490 mm, more than 3 times air saturation. (Jones[106])

adaptations designed to make the most of low or periodic oxygen supply, which will concern us later, are of much avail and a predominantly anaerobic existence is the only one possible. Indeed, here we find most of the organisms which are obligate anaerobes, so adapted to life without oxygen that its presence, even at very low pO_2s, is toxic. Not all intestinal parasites have so far adapted—facultative anaerobes such as the tapeworms can still utilize oxygen when available.*

Environmental carbon dioxide

Some attention must also be given to the carbon dioxide content of the environment. By and large, increases in ambient pCO_2 to the point of serious respiratory inconvenience seldom occur. In aerial environments, despite a somewhat lower diffusion velocity (inversely proportional to square root of molecular weight), gaseous carbon dioxide still diffuses sufficiently rapidly to prevent any significant local accumulations; though in water-logged soils temporary increases up to

* According to Lee and Smith[134] the anaerobic nature of the gut habitat has been exaggerated.

50 mm may occur. There has recently been much concern about the consequences of man's prodigal combustion of fossil fuels but of course the dangers are more likely to arise from climatic changes due to modifying the physical properties of the atmosphere (the so called 'greenhouse effect') than from the direct respiratory consequences of increased pCO_2. In purely local terms the consequences of combustion (both organic and inorganic) are minimal; thus in urban streets a swing of about 0.05% and in crowded indoor situations of up to 1% in the proportions of oxygen and carbon dioxide are of no respiratory consequence.[128]

In aquatic environments the picture is complicated by the presence of buffer systems, so that quite large quantities of carbon dioxide may be present at very low tensions due to the formation of bicarbonates. Such environmental buffer systems are especially well marked in sea-water where in spite of very high carbon dioxide contents, pCO_2 rarely departs appreciably from the atmospheric equilibrium value of 0.23 mm.

Fresh waters usually have much lower buffering capacities (alkali reserve) but even if all the oxygen in an enclosed volume of initially air-saturated distilled water were converted to carbon dioxide by processes of aerobic metabolism, the pCO_2 would not rise above 5 mm because of the very high solubility of this gas (p. 4). It is under conditions favouring intensive anaerobic fermentation that high aqueous pCO_2s are liable to occur; in the papyrus swamps, already referred to, pCO_2 values as high as 35 mm have been recorded.[27,109]

The general tendency for ambient pCO_2 to remain low and constant in aquatic environments and hence in contact with gill epithelia is in marked contrast to the possibility of pCO_2 variation within lung cavities. This contrast is reflected in the arrangements for respiratory regulation which are discussed later (p. 149).

5 The Demand for Oxygen

The arrangements necessary to satisfy an animal's need for oxygen are related to the magnitude of its energy requirements. While in all animals energy can be derived to a greater or lesser degree from anaerobic processes, there is apparently an enormous advantage to be gained in almost all cases, from a maximal use of aerobic processes (p. 2). A review of the variety and complexity of respiratory adaptations (which are in reality principally oxygen exploiting adaptations) furnishes a clear demonstration of the importance of this advantage.

It is interesting to note that in most discussions of respiration, it is tacitly assumed that oxygen consumption gives a full measure of metabolic rate; clearly this is only true if oxygen supply is not limiting and it is perhaps an indication of our faith in the adequacy of respiratory adaptations that we do not more often qualify this assumption. Before proceeding to an examination of the adaptations themselves, it is useful to look at some of the factors on which the demand for oxygen depends.

SIZE

We saw in Chapter 2 that for a given metabolic rate it is possible to define in a general way the maximum size of an organism for which certain levels of gas exchange provision would be adequate. This theoretical approach overlooks the fact that metabolism (measured as oxygen uptake per unit time) is not simply proportional to size; if it were, uptake per unit weight and unit time should be

Table 5.1 Basal metabolism and body weight in rodents. All measurements as oxygen consumption (ml/kg/hr) at air temperatures between 24° and 28°C. (From Bishop[19] and Prosser[174])

	Weight (g)	BMR		Weight (g)	BMR
Long-tailed shrew	3.4	13.7	White mouse	21.2	1.59
Wandering shrew	4.5	8.6	Red-backed mouse	22.8	1.50
Monterey shrew ♂	6.7	7.2	Deer mouse	24.2	1.46
Sonoma shrew ♂	9.2	6.1	Pine mouse	26.3	2.56
Sonoma shrew ♀	11.2	5.5	Dormouse	43.0	1.75
Harvest mouse	9.6	3.8	Hamster	100.0	1.05
Kangaroo mouse ♂	14.4	3.7	Ground squirrel	227.0	0.95
Kangaroo mouse ♀	14.8	3.4	White rat	282.0	0.88
House mouse	15.8	1.53	Guinea pig	460.0	0.76
Deer mouse	17.1	1.65	Hedgehog	684.0	0.74

constant for similar animals of different sizes. In fact it is quite clear from consideration of Table 5.1 that with increasing size in a group of similar animals, oxygen consumption declines.

Rubner[189] is usually credited with the first investigation of the basal metabolism/size relationship. In his study of a variety of breeds of dog, he found that oxygen uptake was in fact proportional to the two-thirds power of body weight ($W^{2/3}$), which represents a fairly close measure of surface area. This sort of relationship holds within all warm-blooded species which have been investigated and is also true to a fair degree for a mixed group of warm-blooded species (Fig. 5.1). Rubner and others suggested that basal metabolism was related to conditions of heat loss as governed by surface area. This overlooks the fact that in many forms much heat is lost from the lungs which are not always included in the surface area estimate. On the other hand, in hibernating mammals in which temperature regulation is abandoned, it has been claimed that oxygen uptake does become proportional to weight[114] (but see p. 26). The tendency for

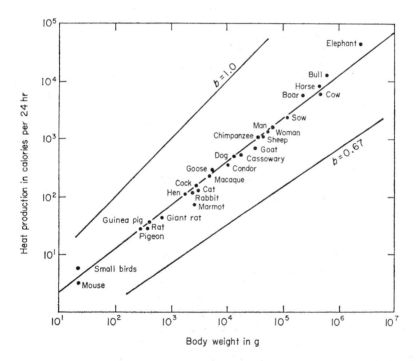

Fig. 5.1 Relationship between total metabolism and body weight in homoiothermic animals. In the double logarithmic plot, the value of the exponent b in the metabolism/ body weight equation is represented by the slope of the regression line through the points—here drawn as 0.75; the lines representing proportionality of metabolism to body weight ($b = 1.0$) and to surface area ($b = 0.67$) are given for comparison. (After Benedict[16])

metabolism to reflect surface area rather than body weight was subsequently found to be equally characteristic of many cold-blooded groups (both vertebrate and invertebrate) so some other explanation is required.

Weight exponent in metabolism

The metabolism/weight relationship can be expressed by the simple exponential formula:

$$M = kW^b \text{ or } \log M = \log k + b \log W$$

where M is oxygen uptake in unit time, W is body weight, k and b are constants. It follows that in the case of any group of animals for which k and b have common values, a plot of log M against log W will give a straight line whose slope is defined by the exponent b and which intercepts the ordinate at k. When b is 1, metabolism is simply proportional to weight but in almost every carefully investigated case b is found to be less than 1. The value which best fits all mammals is 0.75, compared with an exponent of 0.67 for surface area (Fig. 5.1). In the literature may be found values, obtained with various kinds of animal groups (inter- and intra-specific), ranging from 0.45 to 1 but most cases are met by values of 0.7 or over. In assessing the value of b it is important within any experimental group of a single species, to attempt to separate size variation from age variation because the latter may itself be an important factor influencing metabolic rate.

Many parameters have been proposed as determinants of b including organic nitrogen content; abundance of mitochondria, cytochrome oxidase or cytochrome c. Attempts have also been made to relate values of b to such features as growth patterns; type of respiratory exchange mechanism; changes in enzyme concentrations or active/inactive tissue proportions.[174, 238, 239] It is possible that the diversity of exact values of b will be found to reflect a similar diversity of determinants.

Reviewing a wide range of data on the metabolism/body weight relationship, Zeuthen[238] concluded that, considering the whole range of sizes of organisms, metabolism passes through three phases. For small unicellular forms (including bacteria, protozoa and some marine eggs) the exponent b is about 0.7; in the weight range from about 1 μg to 40 mg b increases to about 0.95; finally, above 40 mg a value of about 0.75 is found. Poikilotherms and homoiotherms give lines of the same slope but the latter is at a higher level (cf. Fig. 5.3). In the phylogeny of animals, Zeuthen thus saw a three-phase development, the middle one providing, at the point where metazoan organization began to emerge, a transition to a higher level of metabolism. He sees the evolution of metazoa as essential to phylogenetic increase in size because even if the problems of large single cell organization could have been overcome, very large single-celled organisms would inevitably have had an abysmally low metabolic rate. Similarly, the emergence of homiothermy demanded the stepping-up of metabolism onto a still higher plane, because the poikilotherms were likewise 'running out of steam' as they got bigger. On the basis of data from only four species, Zeuthen further proposed that in this respect ontogeny recapitulates phylogeny, it being claimed that in development from the egg, through the larval, to the adult forms a similar three-phase sequence was found for *Mytilus, Artemia, Asterias* and *Rana.* He suggested that the elevation of metabolism in early homoiothermic forms, resulted from a great extension of the transition phase, so that the relationship would level-off again to a slope of 0.75 at a higher level than in poikilotherms. A somewhat different interpretation of these points is given below.

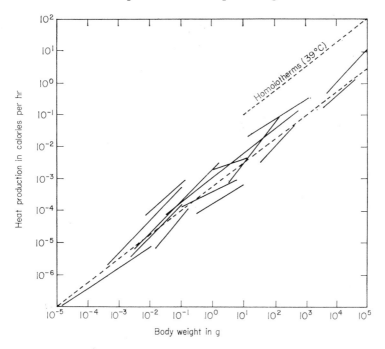

Fig. 5.2 A selection of 'short range lines' relating log. metabolism to log. body weight for a variety of poikilotherms and corrected to a standard temperature of 20°C. Each line represents the variation within a group of closely related animals or a single species. The broken line is the standard poikilotherm line based on earlier data selected by Krogh for their determination under rigorous basal conditions at a temperature of 20°C. The homoiotherm line (cf. Fig. 5.3) for observations corrected to 39°C, is given for comparison. The selection of 15 lines from Hemmingsen's total of 50, has been made for the sake of clarity but does include all the more extreme deviations from the standard line. Metabolism is expressed in Calories/hr but in almost all cases the values were calculated from gas exchange measurements.

Taken in ascending order of minimum weight, the individual lines relate to: various insect eggs (an exception to the normal unicellular line); various adult Diptera; various brackish and freshwater gastropods; various adult Coleoptera; various tropical and arctic insects; leeches, *Glossiphonia* and *Erpobdella*; various crustacea; frogs, *Hyla* and *Pseudacris*; *Ascaris*; killifish, *Fundulus*; eel, *Anguilla*; carp, *Cyprinus*; lungfish, *Protopterus*; various snakes; various tortoises (less shell). (After Hemmingsen[82])

Re-interpretation of weight exponents

Hemmingsen[82] more recently has made a critical examination and assessment of an enormous range of data published in this field. He corrected many earlier measurements of gas exchange to a common temperature (20°C for poikilotherms and 39°C for homoiotherms) and examined the statistical significance of many of the published values of the metabolism/weight exponent b (by him designated n). His conclusion was that with the possibility of a short transition region (0.1 μg to 0.1 mg) where b may approach 1, the value of 0.75 is universal. Most deviations from this value, if not attributable to lack of rigour in defining and establishing truly basal metabolism, are of very limited extent, i.e. restricted to animals within a short range of body weights. The standard log. metabolism/ log. body weight line (of slope 0.75) for poikilotherms was based on the most careful measurements on some 10 species at 20°C selected by Krogh ([123] p. 145). When those later data which are sufficiently reliable, are corrected for temperature (using Krogh's curve (Fig. 5.4), the lines for individual groups are found to lie scattered about the standard line in random fashion; some lie above, others lie below; some are more and others are less steep (Fig. 5.2). Hemmingsen considers that more rigorous control of basal conditions would bring some of these lines more into conformity with the standard. Where real deviations exist they are restricted and so indicate a definite limit to the tolerable departure from the universal norm.

The exponent b appears to have the same value (0.75) for homoiotherms and for unicellular organisms (with yeasts added to the list of forms considered by Zeuthen) but in these cases the values of k in the metabolism/body weight equation are different, so that the lines for these types lie respectively above and below (but parallel to) the poikilotherm standard (Fig. 5.3). In a general way the higher level of the poikilotherm and homoiotherm metabolism, compared with that of unicellular (spherical) forms, is supported by an increased body surface (departure from spherical shape) plus the development of respiratory organs. It can also be shown for insects, birds and mammals that the metabolism required for maximal sustained work is probably also proportional to the same (0.75) power of the body weight. It is of considerable interest that larger flying insects attain body temperatures similar to those of homoiotherms and that the metabolism/weight line for maximum work in larger flying insects (blowfly, horse-fly, butterfly, bee and locust) is continuous with the elevated line for working homoiotherms (Fig. 5.3, see also p. 33). Conversely, the metabolism/weight line in hibernating mammals still has a slope of 0.75 but drops to the level of the standard poikilotherm line. This fall is much greater than would be expected simply on the basis of the reduced body temperature.

Significance of the weight exponent

In an earlier paper Hemmingsen[81] discusses some of the theoretical problems which would arise if metabolism did increase in direct proportion to body weight (i.e. $b = 1$). To take an example from the fishes—if the smallest known fish, *Schindleria* with an adult weight of about 2 mg (2.10^{-3} g), were scaled up to the size of a giant shark at about 10 tons (10^7 g) with metabolism increased in direct proportion, it would have to dissipate about 400 times as much heat as it would if metabolism increased as the 0.75 power of the body weight. Such a rate of heat dissipation would probably mean the raising of the temperature of the water passing over the gills by about 10°C. Similarly, if a rat of 100 g were scaled up to

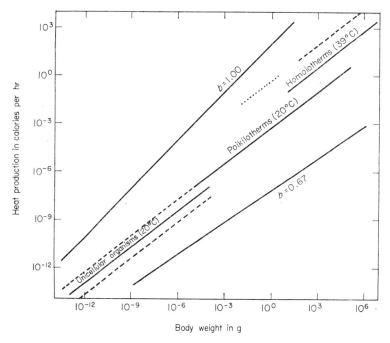

Fig. 5.3 Standard energy metabolism lines, relating log. metabolism to log. body weight, for unicellular organisms (including bacteria, yeasts, protozoa and various marine eggs), poikilotherms and homoiotherms. Metabolic rates corrected (where necessary) to the standard temperatures indicated. In each case the line has been assumed to have a slope (*b*) of 0.75 but its height above the abscissa has been determined by the best fit to the data in the literature. Lines of slope 1.00 (metabolism proportional to weight) and 0.67 (metabolism proportional to surface area) are given for comparison. The extent to which the exponent 0.75 fits the experimental data can be estimated by comparison with Fig. 5.1 (for homoiotherms) and Fig. 5.2 (for poikilotherms). The data for unicellular organisms show a relatively greater scatter (roughly indicated by the broken lines) but there seems to be no reason to propose a line of a different slope and the difference in height between this line and the poikilotherm line is probably highly significant; it has been proposed that there is a transition phase ($b = 1$) between the two lines, in the weight range 10^{-6} to 10^{-3} g. The broken and dotted lines at top right represent maximal sustained work in homoiotherms and larger flying insects respectively (smaller flying insects do not depart significantly from the standard poikilotherm line). (After Hemmingsen[82])

B

the weight of a medium sized elephant of 3 tons (3.10^6 g), the skin temperature of the latter would have to be maintained at about 130°C in order to dissipate the heat produced. Hemmingsen calculates that the maximum weight of a rat is in fact of the order of 350 g if b is 1 and body temperature is not to be raised. Extrapolation of surface-dependent absorptive functions leads to similar absurdities. It is well understood that the lower limit on the size of birds and mammals is governed by the time available for feeding in order to maintain body temperature; in both cases the limit is about 3.5 g (humming birds and long-tailed shrew).

Hemmingsen[82] also has some very interesting speculations about the evolutionary consequences of his conclusions on metabolism/body weight relations. He is unable to accept that, already at the smallest microscopic sizes of unicellular organisms, some allometric relationship was established which subsequently proved capable of sustaining surface area (and cross-section) dependent functions satisfactorily in the largest metazoa. Instead, he postulates a system of 'ortho-selection' (rather than orthogenesis) continuously promoting the preservation of an adaptive trend. With increasing size in any group, metabolism has constantly had to adapt (through natural selection) to the structural necessities, not least to those of the surface-dependent functions. This would account for the limited size range of any departures from the normal exponent of 0.75 (Fig. 5.2). It remains to account for the 'universality' of 0.75 rather than 0.67, which more strictly reflects surface area relations. Hemmingsen's tentative suggestion is that in the course of evolution of the size of animals there has been constantly a tendency for metabolism to increase in proportion to size (i.e. without restraint) and that this trend has been in conflict with surface-dependent limitations. An exponent of about 0.75 may therefore represent a compromise between the trend and the limitations—an indication of the extent to which a group evolving towards greater size can ignore the consequences of surface relationships.

Weight exponent in isolated tissues

Finally, it should be emphasized that the approximate dependence of metabolic rate on the surface area of the body is not simply a reflection of limitations on the rate of entry of oxygen. This is evident from the fact that all animals are capable of great increases over the basal rate (see below), which we have been discussing, but it is also borne out by some observations on the metabolism of isolated tissues. Even when oxygen uptake is measured for tissue slices, the livers of rat, rabbit and sheep show a systematic decrease with increasing body weight and the body weight exponent proves to be 0.75.[117]

Krebs[119] found in a wide range of animals a general tendency for the Qo_2 of isolated tissues of larger animals to be lower than that of the smaller but the tissue Qo_2 changes much less with body weight than does basal metabolism. In a series of mammals (mouse, rat, dog) most of the twelve tissues tested showed a decreasing rate of metabolism but not in strict proportion to the decrease in total metabolism.[152] In other cases, for example a variety of fish organs, tissue metabolism does not correlate with any exponent of body size.[212] Some attempts have been made to summate the metabolism of individual organs and tissues.[152] These do not equate with the metabolism of the whole animal; for the mouse the sum is 72% of the whole; for the dog 106%.

AGE AND DEVELOPMENT

Even after allowing for variation in size there remain some correlations between metabolism and ontogenetic development. For example, in a comparison of three men aged 15, 24 and 71 years, all of whom had approximately the same surface area, oxygen uptake rates of 298, 272 and 205 ml/kg/hr respectively were found ([80] p. 263). A common pattern is of a low basal rate in early larval or foetal growth, rising to a peak sometime in late development and followed by an irregular decline with further ageing. In man the peak is at about the time of natural weaning (3 years), in rats, cattle and pigs sometime between weaning and puberty but in horses not until maturity.[24] The age decline of metabolism per unit area in man is steepest between about 7 and 12 years; a partial arrest occurs during adolescence, especially in boys, followed by a further rapid drop to the age of about 21, when a final phase of slow but steady decline begins and persists throughout the rest of the life. This relates to the problem of hypothermia in old age. At all stages, beyond the 3-year peak, there is a slightly lower rate (even allowing for the size difference) in females than in males.[42] Similar sex differences have been found in other vertebrates, including rats, chickens and snakes.[31]

Metabolic rate increases may also be related to particular events in embryonic development e.g. at fertilization (sea urchin, *Arbacia*; killifish, *Fundulus*) or at the end of gastrulation (*Rana*). In holometabolous insects there is commonly a gradual increase during larval development which is interrupted by a sudden drop early in pupal life and followed by a sharp rise just before emergence. In hemimetabolous insects there is characteristically a rise just after each moult and a decline during the intermoult. For references to these and other examples from invertebrates the reader should consult the textbook of Prosser and Brown.[174]

TEMPERATURE

The influence of temperature on metabolic rate has been one of the most widely studied relationships in the whole domain of respiratory physiology. Many unsuccessful attempts have been made to systematize the results in terms of some relatively simple and universal mathematical functions, such as the van't Hoff or Arrhenius equations, in order to shed light on the controlling mechanisms. The difficulties arise from the mistaken application of these simple principles to processes which essentially proceed in complex chains and there has been much discussion of the role of master reactions. A review of this topic is outside the scope of the present work since the problem is really one of internal control of metabolism. Readers interested in this field should consult the reviews of Bělehrádek[15] and Barnes.[11]

So far as the present discussion is concerned, we may recall that it is often useful to specify the extent of increase in the rate of any function with rise in temperature in the form of a value of Q_{10}:

$$Q_{10} = \frac{K_1^{10/t_1 - t_2}}{K_2}$$

where K_1 and K_2 may be taken, in the present context, as rates of oxygen consumption at the corresponding temperatures t_1 and t_2 (°C). Commonly and especially as regards oxygen consumption, values of Q_{10} vary in different parts of the temperature range (Table 5.2).

Krogh[123] found that the temperature relations of oxygen consumption in a wide range of animals could be expressed by a single curve (Fig. 5.4). This curve has often been used by later workers (e.g. by Hemmingsen—see p. 26) to correct

Table 5.2 Variation of Q_{10} with temperature. Values in the centre column derive from Krogh's classic curve for frogs, fishes and dog (see Fig. 5.4); those in the right-hand column from his work on *Tenebrio* pupae. (Krogh[123])

Temperature range (°C)	Q_{10} for fishes etc.	Q_{10} for *Tenebrio*
0 – 5	10.9	—
5 –10	3.5	—
10 –15	2.9	5.7
15 –20	2.5	3.3
20 –25	2.2	2.6
25 –27.5	2.2	2.3
27.5–30	—	2.1
30 –32.5	—	2.0

observations made at a variety of temperatures to a common standard for comparative purposes. This procedure, though convenient, is no doubt erroneous in some cases because Krogh's curve is not of precise universal application. For example, in the case of *Tenebrio* pupae (meal worms) the curve rises more steeply. This is tantamount to saying that the Q_{10} does not vary uniformly with temperature in all animals (Table 5.2).

Krogh's curve includes values of oxygen consumption for a curarized dog, which illustrate the fact that even for homoiotherms, if subject to artificial variation in body temperature, the same kind of temperature/metabolism relation holds; indeed in this case the dog values fit the curve as well as those of any of the poikilotherms (Fig. 5.4). However, in normal homoiotherms a fall

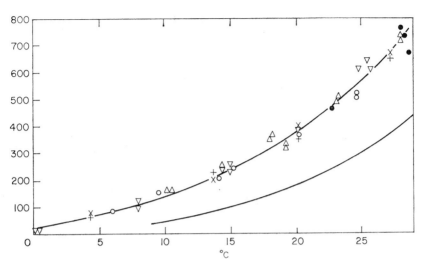

Fig. 5.4   Variation of basal metabolic rate with temperature. The upper curve describes the relationship for: × decerebrate toad; + narcotized and o curarized frogs; ∇ normal and Δ narcotized goldfish; ● curarized dog. The ordinal values for oxygen uptake have been reduced to a common arbitrary standard. The lower curve is for *Tenebrio* pupae—the ordinal values in this case are in ml/kg/hr; reducing these to the common standard would give a curve appreciably steeper than the common curve. (After Krogh[123])

in ambient temperature below the limit of thermal neutrality, causes an increase in metabolic activity as aspects of so-called chemical temperature regulation come into play (e.g. shivering). Above the thermo-neutral zone, physical regulation may succeed in keeping body temperature at the normal level, up to a point beyond which oxygen consumption will rise.

The matter of temperature/metabolism relations is further complicated by the whole question of acclimation and acclimatization to other than 'normal' temperatures for particular species. This is true for both poikilotherms and homoiotherms. Accordingly the greatest caution must be exercised in comparing oxygen uptake rates for animals artificially or naturally exposed to different ambient temperatures. Again we are in danger of straying beyond the proper confines of the present work but the reader may consult the textbook of Prosser and Brown[174] for references in this field.

ACTIVITY

The factors so far considered as modifiers of the demand for oxygen do not, in normal circumstances, call in question the capability of the respiratory organs and circulatory system to deliver adequate quantities of oxygen, though the combined effects of temperature on metabolic rate and solubility of oxygen in the medium may present problems for aquatic poikilotherms (p. 16). The respiratory system is put to a severe test in meeting the needs of high levels of activity.

The maximum level of activity in any animal must, in the last analysis, depend on the body temperature and the upper limit set by this factor on the rate of necessary chemical and physical events within the cell. This is well illustrated by the lethargy of poikilotherms at low ambient temperatures. It is well known that lizards and some insects, for example locusts, orientate to the sun in such a way as to increase heat absorption in the early part of the day and to minimize absorption as the sun gets higher. A further example of the importance of body temperature in limiting activity is found in the warming-up activities of some insects (e.g. butterflies) and waking bats, which are a necessary prelude to flight. Even in man maximal sustained activity is only achieved with a rise in body temperature of about 2°C above the normal. Within the limits set by temperature, vertebrates and probably the more active invertebrates can reach very high levels of activity for short periods, which are considerably in excess of the capacity of the respiratory system to deliver oxygen. They do this simply by going into oxygen debt, a feature which will be discussed later (p. 155). In such short-burst activity, where limitations of oxygen supply are overridden, muscle viscosity may be the limiting factor.

Maximal sustained activity is normally considerably lower than the maximal short-burst level (because the total oxygen debt is strictly limited) and this lower limit is directly dependent on the capacity for oxygen delivery. Both short-burst and sustained activity metabolism have been intensively studied in man, in relation to athletic performance and much is known about the effects of training on improvement of the capacity of the respiratory system, oxygen debt tolerance etc.[7,158]

Upper limits of activity

Whereas the short-burst maximum in man and in the horse exceeds the basal metabolic rate by a factor of about 100, the maximal oxygen uptake in sustained muscular activity is limited to about 20 times the basal level in both species. For an activity level which can be sustained for long periods, such as a working day, the factor falls to between 3 and 8 in both cases. It is interesting that these ratios are independent of body weight over a tenfold range—68 kg for man, 680 kg for the horse.[40]

The metabolic rate of 'resting' humming-birds is about 4 times what would be expected from Hemmingsen's homoiotherm line (Fig. 5.3)—because of nervousness and restlessness basal conditions cannot be achieved without narcosis. The metabolism of hovering humming-birds is about 6 times the 'resting' level, so again there is at least a twentyfold increase over the presumed basal level (Pearson[168] quoted by Hemmingsen[82]). On the basis of measured basa rates and calculated rates for flying speeds of 53 to 63 km per hr, Hemmingsen[82] finds the maximal/basal ratio to lie between 20 and 33 for the pigeon.

He also calculates that for dogs on a treadmill the maximal/basal ratio is about 18.

Hemmingsen has also reviewed a wide range of studies on flying insects and here the maximal/basal ratios seem to fall into two groups. In larger forms (blowfly, horse-fly, bee, butterfly and locusts) ranging from 31 mg to 1.8 g, body temperature increases during sustained flight to a level typical of homoiotherms. Under these conditions maximal sustained metabolism is as much as 575 times the basal level. From observations on smaller insects (*Drosophila*, *Simulium* and *Aëdes*) with a weight range from 0.9 to 8.1 mg, the maximal/basal ratio lies much closer to that for homoiotherms but has not been precisely determined. It is thought that these small insects are unable to sustain a body temperature much above ambient during flight.

6 The Circulation

For a more or less spherical animal in excess of 1 mm diameter, some sort of internal convection or circulatory system is necessary for the maintenance of a reasonable metabolic rate (p. 6). This helps to overcome the limitation of the slowness of diffusion of the respiratory gases through the tissues and will give an adequate backing to diffusion through the general body surface up to the size of a sphere about 1 cm in diameter. Beyond this point, the circulation must be associated with specialized surfaces for gas exchange (p. 7). These size limits must be interpreted flexibly and in both cases some exceptions have already been noted (Chapter 2).

TYPES OF CIRCULATORY SYSTEM

The circulation of body fluids serves many purposes besides gas transport but fulfilment of this particular function undoubtedly dictates the rate at which the circulation proceeds. Some kinds of slowly circulating body fluids (e.g. intercellular or tissue fluid and lymph), on the other hand, are not significantly concerned in gas transport, so our concern is restricted to blood and/or coelomic fluid. Propulsion of these fluids is, with only one or two exceptions, dependent in one form or another on muscular activity. This is not an appropriate place for a detailed review of the vascular anatomy of the various groups (for which the review of Martin and Johansen[152] and the standard vertebrate texts may be consulted); attention will be confined to a summary of some of the more general principles as they affect respiratory function.

Coelomic circulation

Beyond the streaming movements of protoplasm, which undoubtedly do enhance intracellular diffusion processes, the most elementary kind of internal circulation of respiratory significance is that found in the pseudocoel of nematodes. Here, as in the true coelom of sipunculids, echiuroids, polychaetes and holothurians, the contents of a relatively extensive cavity are gently mixed by contractions of the body wall musculature and there is in no sense a directional system of circulation. This simple churning up of a fluid which bathes the inside of the respiratory surface and the outside of masses of respiring tissues, nevertheless, contributes substantially to the net gas flux into and out of the body. The frequent presence of respiratory pigments in such fluids bears witness to a respiratory function, though as we shall see later (p. 140) it does not necessarily attest to a transport function *per se*.

Closed vascular systems

At the other extreme of circulatory complexity is the closed vascular system, a complete closed-circuit of narrow blood vessels (of mesodermal origin) enclosing a highly specialized fluid, which alone properly deserves the name of blood. One or more specialized muscular regions (hearts) of this tubular system carry out the main propulsive function, though the arteries, which perform the primary stage of distribution of blood to the tissues, may have subsidiary muscular regulating functions. Significant gas exchange is confined to a more or less well-developed system of very fine, very thin-walled capillaries which ramify through the active tissues. Blood returns to the heart and respiratory surface via larger, usually non-contractile veins. Such completely closed systems are found in many polychaetes and all other annelids, nemerteans, cephalopod molluscs and vertebrates. The blood may pool in localized sinuses or lacunae but such enlargements are morphologically part of the mesodermal vascular system and the endothelial lining is continuous. In a few cases only, the capillary endothelium is absent locally (e.g. in mammalian spleen and the maternal side of the placenta in primates, bats and rodents[160]) and the tissues are actually bathed in blood.

The pressure required to circulate blood through such a closed system is high and if the propulsive power is confined to a single heart, as in vertebrates, it consists of several chambers in series. In fishes a single circuit embraces the gills and the tissues, with the heart preceding the gills. Cephalopod molluscs have paired subsidiary branchial hearts, which pump the blood through the highly developed gills, while the heart proper, filling with oxygenated blood via paired atria, has a single ventricle driving blood into the general body circulation.[102] There is conflicting evidence about the contractility of other parts of the vascular system.[86] With the emergence of alveolar lungs in the higher vertebrates, blood pumped by the heart through the lung capillary system returns to that organ and being kept partly separated (in amphibia and reptiles) or completely separated (in the homoiotherms) from incoming venous blood, is passed to the tissues by a second propulsive effort. The cardiovascular system of tunicates is unique. It consists essentially of an exceptionally thin-walled heart, pumping blood alternately out of either end into a system of 'arteries' and capillaries which open into tissue spaces. Periodically, the heart beat is reversed so that blood is sucked back via the same vessels now acting as 'veins'.[155] Increasing the pressure in the arteries by as little as 0.1 mm is sufficient to cause the reversal of contraction.[121]

Although the characteristic vascular system of polychaetes is closed, in some forms it is reduced or rudimentary (e.g. in Glyceridae, Capitellidae and *Polycirrus*) and the coelomic fluid, assisted by muscular movements of the body wall, assumes an important role in distributing oxygen. Even in the case of polychaetes with a well-developed closed system, the coelomic fluid probably contributes because of the poor capillary development (p. 134). Many invertebrates show, by vertebrate standards, poor development of tissue capillaries. This deficiency is probably offset by a number of factors, including lower metabolic rate; greater tolerance of anaerobiosis; and in certain situations, diffusion facilitation by myoglobins (p. 135).

Open vascular systems

Functionally intermediate between the random-mixing coelomic system and the completely closed circulation, lie a number of types known as 'open' vascular systems. However, the openness is a matter of degree and no absolute line of distinction can be drawn even between the open and closed types. Nevertheless, the open systems have certain features in common: a single muscular heart propels blood through a branching arrangement of arteries and capillaries from which it emerges into a system of larger (sinus) or smaller (lacuna) spaces, known as the haemocoel, which are remnants of the primary body cavity (blastocoel). The endothelial linings of these spaces are incomplete so that the blood, usually called 'haemolymph',* bathes the tissues directly. In the non-cephalopod molluscs, blood is returned from the haemocoelic spaces to the heart via a well-defined system of contractile veins, traversing the capillary system of the respiratory organ on the way—only the renal blood misses the respiratory organ. The heart is slightly built but divided into two chambers—atrium and ventricle.

Arthropod blood is returned to the heart in a somewhat different manner. In decapod crustacea, for example, all the blood from the sinus system passes through the gills and is then disgorged into an extensive dorsal sinus which surrounds the pericardium (attached in the dorsal mid-line to the underside of the carapace); thence it passes via a series of openings into the pericardium and via the valved ostia into the heart itself.[26] The heart has a single chamber and there are no veins. The insect circulatory system differs from that of the crustacea in having (a) many contractile arteries and (b) no significant respiratory function.

Echinoderms, other than holothurians, have an essentially open system in which all the body fluid systems (except the ambulacral) are in communication with each other in varying degrees. In the water-vascular system the circulation is due to ciliary action. Unlike those of arthropods and molluscs, this open system probably does not exhibit overall a well defined unidirectional flow.

CIRCULATORY FACTORS

In considering the efficacy of circulatory systems, especially in regard to their most exacting gas transport function, a number of parameters are of importance.

---

* The term 'haemolymph' is open to objection, since the fluid in question does not combine the roles of vertebrate blood and lymph. It does, however, combine the functions of blood and interstitial fluid, forming the internal milieu of most invertebrates.

Principally these are gas capacity, blood volume, flow rate and pressure. The capacity for carrying oxygen and carbon dioxide will be considered in detail in later chapters but the other factors will now be considered briefly.

Blood volume

Blood volume may be estimated by a number of sophisticated techniques but a simple approximation (usually giving minimal values) may be obtained by bleeding plus estimation of residual blood after maceration and extraction. Some methods measure total extracellular space—i.e. including tissue fluid and lymph. Collections of values and descriptions of the methods may be found in various textbooks.[172,173] It should be noted that while values for animals with closed systems are generally low, those for animals with open systems are much higher since in this case haemolymph occupies virtually the whole of the total extracellular space. Some representative values are given in Table 6.1. The majority of

Table 6.1 Representative values for blood volume in ml/100 g of body weight; for closed circulatory systems unless otherwise indicated: * open systems or † purely coelomic systems. Where a range is given, higher values are probably more reliable as in most cases these are based on more exact methods (e.g. dye dilution). Values in brackets for closed systems represent total extracellular fluid compartment, determined by a dilution method using inulin, thiocyanate or radio-isotope. (From data collected by Prosser[172, 173])

Man	6.2–7.0 (17.5)	*Petromyzon*	8.5 (18.5)
Dog	6.2–10.5	*Octopus*	5.8 (28.0)
Goat	6.1–7.3	*Achatina* *	40.4
Rat (albino)	5.7	*Planorbis* *	30.0–58.1
Rabbit	4.3–6.5	*Aplysia* *	79
Pigeon	7.8	*Mytilus* *	50.8
Chicken	7 (♀)–9 (♂)	*Mazaritana* * (F. W. bivalve)	49
Turtle	7.4	*Cambarus* *	25.1–25.6
Alligator	4.2	*Homarus* *	17.0
Rana pipiens	8.0 (27.3)	*Maia* * (hard)	8–15
Rana temporaria	4.6	(fresh moulted)	29–70
Ameirus (teleost)	1.8 (4.0)	*Bombyx* * (larva)	28.6–31.2
Anguilla	2.9	*Periplaneta* * (adult)	19.5
Squalus	6.8–8.7 (12.7)	*Sipunculus*†	50
Raja	4.6	*Urechis*†	33

vertebrates show much the same blood volume ranging between about 6 and 10% of the body weight but on the basis of a rather limited number of observations, the values for teleosts seem to be significantly lower (< 3). It is claimed that relative blood volume decreases with increase in body size in mammals (cf. O_2 uptake and body weight—p. 23).[72] Cephalopod blood volumes are similar to those of vertebrate closed systems (so are the extracellular fluid volumes) and in marked contrast to the higher values found in the open systems, which include extracellular space, of the other molluscan groups. The blood volumes of the arthropod open systems are intermediate.

It can hardly be doubted that where a premium is put on the rate of uptake and distribution of oxygen, a rapid circulation of a relatively small amount of blood within a closed system is more efficient than the sluggish circulation of a much larger volume which meanders through all the extracellular space. The closure of the cephalopod system is an apt adaptation to high activity, while the most active arthropods, the insects, do not use their open vascular system for respiratory purposes. A large, if slowly moving, blood volume may have advantages in other ways, if it can be afforded, e.g. as a store for antibodies, phagocytes, etc. and as a hydrostatic skeleton.[173]

Blood pressure and flow rate

In a closed system, the head of hydrostatic pressure developed by the heart declines with distance from the pump because of internal (viscosity) and external frictional loss and distension of the vessels. The effective force for driving blood between any two points is the difference in blood pressures measured at these two points. The total flow, however, must remain constant at different distances from the heart, though the velocity in individual vessels is roughly inversely proportional to cross-sectional area—in mammals the cross-sectional area of total capillaries is 800 times that of the aorta. Since blood in the larger vessels exhibits laminar flow, the plasma layer in contact with the wall is stationary and velocity increases towards the centre. Consequently, in bloods containing erythrocytes, movement in arteries and veins shows a concentration of the cells in the faster moving central region while the slow moving peripheral layers are cell free. In the capillaries, where gas exchange occurs, the lumen is so narrow that corpuscles often have to be squeezed through and no peripheral stagnation can occur. In bloods without erythrocytes, there may be some tendency still for laminar flow in capillaries and the diffusion barrier, between the vessel and the tissues outside, will then include a thin stationary layer of plasma.

The maximum velocity (V_{max}) between any two points in the system is proportional to the pressure drop (P) and the square of the radius (R) and inversely proportional to viscosity (η); total blood flow (F) follows Poiseuille's Law:

$$V_{max} = \frac{P.R^2}{4\eta} \quad \text{and} \quad F = P \times \frac{\pi}{8} \times \frac{1}{\eta} \times \frac{R^4}{l}$$

The R^4 dependence is particularly important; it means that provided pressure remains constant, blood flow will be halved for only one-sixteenth reduction in radius or diameter or a 50% reduction in diameter will reduce blood flow to one-sixteenth.

Blood pressure measurements, which are made by arresting the flow, give values for the pressure exerted longitudinally in the vessel and these determine flow rates. However, flowing blood also exerts a lateral pressure on the wall of the vessel and tends to distend it. The kinetic energy imparted to the blood by the heart muscle is therefore partly dissipated (in the form of heat) by doing work on the wall of the vessel as well as by frictional losses. If the walls are highly elastic, as in arteries, the distension due to rise in blood pressure at systole tends to be recovered at diastole. The walls then exert a pressure on the blood, which prevented from back flow by the heart valves, is moved forward faster than it would be otherwise at diastole. The elasticity of arteries, therefore, has the effect of spreading or elongating the pulse pressure and so smoothing the flow. Resistance of the walls to distension is much greater in arteries than it is in veins; accordingly, increased flow into an artery increases the pressure markedly, the diameter only moderately, while the reverse is true in veins.

The extensibility and particularly the active contractility of many of the blood vessels complicates the calculation of flow rates because of interconnected changes which occur in the P and R in the Poiseuille formula. Thus, as active contraction of a vessel begins, the slight constriction causes an increase in flow rate due to a rise in pressure. The increased flow is accompanied by a drop in lateral pressure of the blood on the wall and the tension, against which the muscle fibres are working, falls; they therefore shorten further without any increase in muscle tension and further constriction results. Flow rate increases and lateral pressure reduces still further. Very soon, lateral pressure drops below that of the surrounding tissue on the vessel, which collapses completely. The muscle fibres are thus able to shorten maximally and occlude the vessel with minimal effort until they are positively relaxed, e.g. by cessation of nerve impulses or of hormone action.

Regulation of blood flow rate

The contractile nature of vertebrate arteries and arterioles serves to regulate the flow of blood to different parts of the body according to the moment to moment variation in oxygen needs. The principal control of the smooth muscle fibres in the walls of these vessels is by a vasoconstrictor innervation (sometimes also vasodilator) mainly from the autonomic system. Control is also exercised hormonally, especially by the local action of adrenaline, which causes constriction of arterioles. The circulation in particular organs may be controlled additionally by specific hormones, e.g. in the kidney by the renin-angiotensin system. A slight degree of sympathetic vasoconstriction occurs in some veins, at least in mammals. In addition there is the special respiratory significance of arteriolar sensitivity to local pH changes, which are occasioned by rising pCO_2 or concentration of anaerobic acid metabolites. This is an extremely important method of adjustment of supply to demand within different parts of a single organ. It was formerly thought that the capillaries themselves were also independently contractile, due to the presence of scattered muscular cells forming an incomplete second layer outside the endothelium.[127] This view is no longer generally held and the undoubted independent variations of capillary blood flow are usually attributed to the action of scattered contractile cells confined to the outside of the walls of met-arterioles and at arterio-capillary sphincters. Since occlusion at the approach to a capillary reduces the blood pressure within it, the vessel itself will tend to collapse from the pressure of external tissues and give the impression of general capillary constriction.

Resistance to blood flow, which is expressed in arbitrary units, is proportional to the pressure drop between two points and inversely proportional to the volume of blood (cross-section area times distance) contained by the vessel between these points, i.e. $R = (p_1-p_2)/V$. Total resistance is fairly easily determined for a closed system with a single propulsive organ, e.g. in vertebrates. The resistance and the pressure drop are naturally greatest in the capillaries. In mammals, where the systolic/diastolic pressures may be as high as 160/130, the pressure drop along the capillaries may rise as high as 100 mm Hg.

Total blood flow

A further important parameter in haemodynamics is the total blood flow. Again where a single heart is found, blood flow which must equal the cardiac output,

Table 6.2 Some representative values for blood pressure. Normal systolic/diastolic, range of systolic or mean pressures in mm Hg and sites of measurement; * values for hydrostatic pressure in body cavity. (From data collected by Prosser[172, 173] unless otherwise indicated)

Horse	carotid a.	150–194	*Ascidia*		2.0
Cow	carotid a.	125–166	*Homarus*[26]		
Seal	femoral a.	130–150	rest	ventricle	13/1
Man	radial a.	120/80	active	ventricle	27/13
	pulmonary a.	25/8	*Cancer*	ventricle	8
Sheep	carotid a.	90–140	*Maia*	heart	4/3.3
Dog	femoral a.	110	*Octopus*[102]	aorta	33–52
Rhesus			*Helix*	heart	1.1
monkey		159/127	*Lymnaea*	haemo-	
Rabbit	femoral a.	90–100		coel	2.2–8.1
Rat	carotid a.	77	*Anodonta*	heart	4.4
Guinea pig	carotid a.	77/47	*Arenicola*	body	
Stork		161		cavity	26.4
Chicken[207]	carotid a.	142/117	*Lumbricus*	body	
Canary[207]	ventricle	220/154		cavity	10
Crocodile		30–50	*Sipunculus*	coelom	16–71
Pseudemys		42/32	*Ascaris*	pseudo-	
Rana[63]	aorta	15/8		coel	70
Bufo[63]	aorta	26/19	*Holothuria*	body	
Anguilla	v. aorta	25–60		cavity	1.1
Salmo	v. aorta	75	*Caudina*	body	
	d. aorta	53		cavity	29.4
Squalus[25]	v. aorta	39/28			
	d. aorta	30/23			

is readily defined in terms of the stroke volume (times number of beats per minute) or minute volume. However, it is not usually a simple matter to measure cardiac output directly because the necessary surgical procedures tend to alter circulatory performance. Two indirect methods are more reliable. The first is based on an extension of the dye dilution method for blood volume. A known amount of dye (or isotopically labelled compound or erythrocytes) is injected into a vein and the time relations of its recovery in serial samples from an artery are studied. Alternatively, advantage may be taken of the Fick principle, according to which:

$$\text{Cardiac output (l/min)} = \frac{O_2 \text{ consumed (ml/min)}}{\text{arterial} - \text{venous } O_2 \text{ content (ml/l)}}$$

The venous blood content must be determined on mixed venous blood, which is reliably collected only by catheterization of the right ventricle.

Vertebrate and invertebrate haemodynamics

The above discussion of cardiovascular dynamics has largely been condensed from a fuller but still simple treatment by Florey;[51] a more complete account of what has now become an exact science so far as higher vertebrates are concerned,

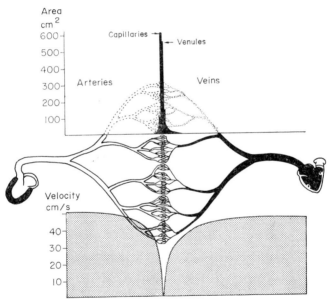

Fig. 6.1 Relationship between total cross-sectional area and blood flow rate at various levels in the circulation of a 13 kg dog. Flow rate at a particular level is inversely proportional to the total area of vessels at that level; the rate in the capillaries is accordingly about one-hundredth that in the larger arteries and veins. (Rushmer[191])

is given by Rushmer.[191] Some of the principal relationships are illustrated in Fig. 6.1.

For invertebrates our knowledge in this field is very incomplete and uneven. The relatively simple haemodynamic principles cease to hold where open circulations are concerned. A good deal is known for invertebrates about the physiology of the heart itself and this has been well summarized by Prosser;[173]

since this aspect does not directly concern our discussion of respiratory function it will not be dealt with here.

Blood pressure of invertebrates

The determination of blood pressure of invertebrates has been widely attempted and some data for comparison with vertebrates are given in Table 6.2. Interest in this field has been concerned among other things with establishing whether or not a sufficient excess of hydrostatic pressure over colloid osmotic pressure is available to effect filtration in invertebrate renal organs.

7 Respiratory Organs

In the development of respiratory organs Nature has been exceptionally inventive. Where the metabolic needs of animals put the demands for oxygen beyond the capacity of the general body surface to admit them, a great diversity of specialized surfaces for respiratory gas exchange has resulted. A broad survey rather than a detailed catalogue will be attempted. For the sake of convenience most of these structures can be placed in two broad categories: (a) evaginated *gills* usually for gas exchange with aquatic media and (b) invaginated *lungs* usually for exchange with the atmosphere. Neither category is absolute and both need to be subdivided.

DUAL EXCHANGE—CUTANEOUS AND RESPIRATORY ORGAN

The development of respiratory organs does not of necessity entirely supersede general surface exchange; the latter may remain to an almost insignificant extent or as in the amphibia, for example, it may continue to play an important part. In all aquatic forms not wholly covered by an impermeable cuticle or shell, some cutaneous exchange is bound to continue and in a few cases its relative importance has been assessed. Where cutaneous and gill exchange occur together in water their respective importance can be roughly estimated by comparison of overall oxygen uptake (and carbon dioxide elimination) with that occurring after extirpation of the gills.

Cutaneous exchange in water

Such experiments have been performed on a number of sabellid polychates. Fox[57] found about 60% reduction of oxygen uptake after amputating the branchial crown of *S. spallanzani*; the crown being itself a very active ciliary feeding structure, in addition to a respiratory organ, this drop may over-estimate the dependence of the rest of the body upon the crown. In *S. pavonina*, on the other hand, Wells[225] found that the total uptake by the two halves of a bisected worm was not significantly lower than that of whole worms, while in *Myxicola infundibulum* there was a sharp drop in total uptake on bisection with the posterior part giving relatively lower values than in *S. pavonina*. This suggests that in the latter species, which irrigates its tube, the crown uptake does not contribute much to the needs of the rest of the body, while in *Myxicola*, which does not irrigate its tube, the whole body is largely dependent on the crown. An assumption that metabolism is normal after the drastic measures of amputation or bisection may not be wholly justified.

A less violent approach to the problem was pursued by Dales.[35] He found in another sabellid, *Schizobranchia insignis*, that crown-amputated worms showed a 75% drop in oxygen consumption, while intact worms prevented from irrigating the tube but with crowns extended had a normal uptake, though they remained extended more continuously than usual. Worms which were allowed to irrigate but prevented from extending the crown showed a 60% drop. These observations still do not permit an exact apportioning of the normal contributions of crown and cutaneous uptake because of possible circulatory and other adaptations to the experimental conditions but they do indicate that potentially the crown alone can supply the whole need and that cutaneous uptake can supply up to 40%. This difference is partly a reflection of the greater rate of irrigation of the branchial crown as measured by actual filtration performance, compared with irrigation of the tube (70 and 12 ml/g/hr respectively) though utilization by the crown is only 10% (cf. other ciliary feeding gills) compared with 24% for the general body surface. If the crown can take up 10% of the oxygen in 70 ml of water while the skin takes up 24% from 12 ml, the crown is more than twice as effective as the skin in actual provision of the animal's needs.

The aquatic pulmonates provide an example of general cutaneous exchange from water complemented by oxygen uptake from the lung. In this case the respective contributions can be separated in simultaneous measurements under something like normal conditions. The situation in *Planorbis* and *Lymnaea* is discussed in detail later (p. 116) but the general position here is one of a highly significant cutaneous uptake with pulmonary function taking over progressively as the dissolved oxygen tension falls.

Cutaneous exchange in air

The third kind of shared function is illustrated by the terrestrial amphibia where both exchanges take place with air. Krogh[122] devised an ingenious method of separating the two aspects in some studies on *Rana*. In *R. fusca* (now *R. temporaria*) mean values of oxygen and carbon dioxide exchange taken between April and October were 52 and 129 ml/kg/hr respectively for the skin and 105 and 45 ml/kg/hr for the lungs. Thus the skin accounts for 33% of oxygen exchange and about 75% of carbon dioxide exchange. Plotting the individual results as a function of time shows an interesting seasonal pattern, which was entirely confirmed by Dolk and Postma[41] for *R. temporaria* (Fig. 7.1). Cutaneous oxygen uptake is almost independent of season, while cutaneous carbon dioxide elimination shows a very pronounced peak during the breeding season. Lung exchange shows a very pronounced peak at this time for both gases. Pulmonary oxygen uptake exceeds cutaneous (with a very marked breeding excess) from March to October but falls short of the cutaneous level during winter hibernation. Carbon dioxide elimination by the lung is much below that of the skin at all times, though both show a similar peak in April. Less extensive data for *R. esculenta*[122] suggests that on average through the year the skin is of even greater relative importance for the exchange of oxygen (50%) and carbon dioxide (86%) than the lungs.

These studies are somewhat suspect because the lungs were ventilated artificially and (in view of the complexity of natural ventilation (p. 59)) possibly

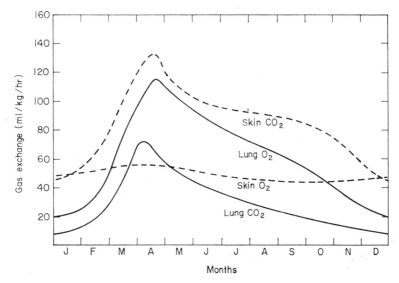

Fig. 7.1 Seasonal change in the pattern of pulmonary and cutaneous gas exchange in *Rana temporaria*. (After Dolk and Postma[41])

abnormally. More recently Whitford and Hutchison ([96] for references) examined the effect of temperature on the dual gas exchange in an extensive range of salamanders, frogs and toads, using a respirometer which permitted natural ventilation. In spite of considerable inter-specific variation, there was a general picture of dominant cutaneous oxygen uptake at lower temperatures with very pronounced increase and eventual dominance of pulmonary uptake at higher temperatures, cutaneous uptake remaining relatively stable. The take over point was generally lower ($< 10°C$) in anurans than in salamanders ($> 13°C$). In the temperate zone anurans, lungs and buccal cavity absorbed about 35% of the oxygen at 5° and about 68% at 25°. Cutaneous carbon dioxide elimination was always dominant (70–95%). Although natural seasonal state was not taken into account, the similarity between the general pattern at temperatures up to 20°C and the January–April part of Dolk and Postma's curve is very striking. Unfortunately, similar comparisons for amphibia immersed in water have not been published but Wolvekamp (personal communication) found in three species of newts (*Triturus*) that while cutaneous uptake alone sufficed out of water, regular lung ventilation was necessary for aquatic life!

Cutaneous and pulmonary capillary systems in Amphibia

Foxon[63] has summarized extensive data on the extent and distribution of the capillary systems concerned with gas exchange in both anurans and urodeles. This provides an alternative but indirect approach to assessing the relative importance of cutaneous and pulmonary oxygen uptake.

In *R. esculenta* the average density of capillary meshes in the whole skin is 220 per mm^2 but on the back and thighs, which are normally well-exposed to the air, the count rises to 300 per mm^2. For inter-specific comparisons estimates of total length of capillaries are more useful. These provide also a basis for rough comparison of the different possible gas exchange sites, i.e. the lungs, the skin and the buccal cavity. Some of the conclusions drawn from such data do not agree precisely with those from direct gas exchange measurements but they do demonstrate some broad generalizations. Thus the proportion of total respiratory capillaries which is found in the lining of the buccal cavity does not exceed 3% except in some lung-less salamanders (Plethodontidae) where the buccal cavity percentage rises to between 5 and 11. In anura the cutaneous capillaries rarely account for more than 50% of the total, whereas in some urodeles (*Triton* spp.) cutaneous capillaries constitute about 75% of the total.

On the alternative basis of length of capillary per gram of body weight, the total respiratory surface figure for *Triton cristatus* is 15.6 m/g and the skin figure is 11.7. By comparison, the total figure for the tree frog *Hyla arborea* is 46.0 m/g and the skin figure is 11.1. Thus the skin capillaries of the relatively inactive and aquatic newt appear capable of subserving three-quarters of its respiratory needs while the same amount of skin capillary can only meet one-quarter of the needs of the more active tree frog.

Adult *Triton cristatus* also exhibit a seasonal variation in skin capillary density. With assumption of the breeding dress the skin capillary count rises very significantly and the newts in water, if deprived of atmospheric oxygen, survive better than non-breeding individuals under the same circumstances.

Foxon concludes that generally uptake of oxygen in the mouth is not significant and the bucco-pharyngeal ventilation probably serves an olfactory function. Exceptionally, significant buccal uptake may occur in the lung-less salamanders and also in *Ambystoma maculatum* in both of which peculiar evaginations of buccal capillaries occur.

It is interesting to recall that in urodeles, where (for at least some forms) cutaneous oxygen exchange is apparently more important than pulmonary exchange, there are no special arrangements for arterial and venous supply to the skin. In anurans, on the other hand, although blood is supplied specifically to the lungs and skin via the pulmo-cutaneous arch, oxygenated blood from the skin returns by way of the sinus venosus to the right atrium and hence becomes mixed with the venous return from the rest of the body. In neither group therefore is the best use made of blood oxygenated in the skin capillaries.

Dominance of respiratory organs

In all these cases cutaneous exchange (particularly of carbon dioxide) looms large and the activity of the specialized respiratory organs is in a sense supplementary. This is doubtless true of many other forms which utilize both skin and gills or lungs. Two factors influencing the structure of the outer body surface swing the balance strongly in favour of the respiratory organs as gas exchangers. These are (a) the need for development of a mechanically robust external skeleton as in arthropods and many echinoderms and (b) need for cuticular impermeability to water in forms which are at odds with the ambient osmotic pressure (notably fishes) or are liable to desiccation (notably reptiles, birds, mammals and land arthropods). In such 'naked' forms as cephalopods, high levels of activity no doubt necessitate a dominance of exchange via the gills. Even when oxygen uptake via respiratory organs assumes a massive dominance, residual exchange through the skin especially of carbon dioxide may still occur to a considerable degree. Thus the cutaneous loss of carbon dioxide as a percentage of pulmonary elimination is 85% in a lizard, 7.6% in the rabbit and 1% in man.[174]

GILLS

Irrigation mechanisms

Gills are found in a great variety of forms and in the great majority of cases some mechanism is present for replenishing the water which bathes their surfaces. This may simply depend on ciliary action as on the branchial crown of sabellids, on the parapodial gills of such errant polychaetes as *Nephtys* or on the elaborate and often very extensive ctenidia of various groups of aquatic molluscs (reviewed by Morton and Yonge[159]) and of ascidians. More commonly some form of muscular activity is responsible for an irrigation current. Peristaltic waves in the body wall musculature, which may pass antero-posteriorly (e.g. *Sabella*) or postero-anteriorly (terebellids), are often employed by tubicolous polychaetes. In other forms simple undulating movements of the body irrigate the burrow, e.g. in *Nereis* and chironomid (midge) larvae. The patterns of behaviour, of which these tubicolous irrigation activities form a part, often set up peculiar conditions for gas exchange and need to be carefully considered in studying respiratory performance—some illustrations of this point will be considered in Chapter 9.

Irrigation by the oscillating movements of specialized appendages is found in a few polychaetes (e.g. *Chaetopterus*) but is almost universal among crustacea. Currents produced in this way, along the outside of the body, may also subserve a feeding function as in *Chirocephalus*, *Artemia* and *Daphnia* or serve for respiration alone as in amphipods (*Gammarus*) and isopods (*Idotea*). In decapod crustacea, probably in relation to greater size, the very extensive gills are virtually completely enclosed by lateral extensions of the carapace (the branchiostegite) and the irrigation current, passing in a predominantly postero-anterior direction, is produced by vibration of the scaphognathites (flattened exopodites of the maxillae) and not of the gills themselves as with the abdominal pleopods of isopods. These and other aspects of crustacean respiration have been reviewed by Lockwood.[143]

Irrigation of cephalopod and fish gills

The most complex muscular arrangements for gill irrigation are found in the pumping arrangements of cephalopod molluscs and fishes. In the former the very muscular mantle chamber is provided with effective inlet and outlet valves, formed by the mantle edge and the funnel respectively. Strong rhythmic contractions cause a pulsating current through the cavity in which the gills are freely suspended. In *Nautilus*, where there are two pairs of gills instead of one, the funnel is the main contractile structure.[68] The irrigation current of cephalopods, which is well known to serve a secondary locomotory function, apparently does not have a counter-current relationship to the branchial blood flow (p. 15).[158, 236]

In fishes the arrangements are even more sophisticated. Here the passage of water through the fine sieve-like arrangement of the gill filaments and lamellae (see below) is effected by two pumps working in series, one either side of the gill resistance. This ensures that the flow of water over the respiratory epithelium is virtually continuous, an important advance over the pulsating flow of the cephalopods. A model of this double pumping mechanism is illustrated in Fig. 7.2. The continuity of flow has been deduced by observations of the pressures in the buccal and opercular chambers which lie on either side of the gills. An early, simple observation by van Dam[36] of continuity of flow in an external tube connecting the two chambers was interpreted as an indication that the pressure is always higher in the buccal than in the opercular chamber. Hughes and Shelton,[92] using sensitive recorders inside the chambers, were able to measure the changing pressures within each chamber with some precision and confirmed the superiority of the buccal pressure during at least 90% of each pumping cycle (Fig. 7.3). The morphological arrangements and functional details will not be elaborated here as they are well summarized in the excellent account of vertebrate respiratory physiology by Hughes.[89]

Essentially similar patterns of pressure change and relationships have been found by Saunders[194] in other fresh water species. Two additional points in his study concern the operation during 'heavy breathing' induced by high pCO_2. The momentary reversal of the pressure differential (see Fig. 7.3) partly or completely disappears and there is a tendency for the opposed tips of the gill filaments to part when the differential is maximal during heavy breathing. The latter point will limit the extent to which the utilization can be maintained at high rates of water flow.

The dual pump arrangement is found in essentially the same form in elasmobranchs. There are a few detailed differences including entry via the spiracle in addition to the mouth and exit by five paired parabranchial cavities instead of by a single pair of opercular cavities. The predominantly higher buccal pressure again ensures a virtually continuous flow over the gill epithelium. Some fishes which swim strongly and almost continuously, do not make active respiratory movements while in motion but, swimming with the mouth permanently open, rely on the ram effect. This is well seen in some sharks but the mackerel has gone so far as to lose the power of active irrigation and must swim continuously to

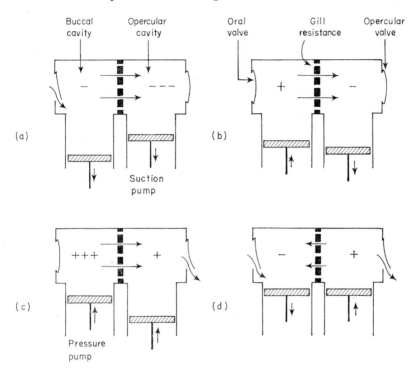

Fig. 7.2 Model of the double pumping mechanism for irrigation of the gills in teleosts and elasmobranchs. The pressures in the buccal and opercular cavities (indicated by + or −) are relative to the water outside. The principal phases are (a) and (c), when water is forced through the gill resistance by suction pumping and pressure pumping respectively. The transition phases (b) and (d) each occupy only about 10% of the duration of the whole cycle. There is a potential reversal of flow during phase (d), due to the momentary reversal of pressure difference but the inertia of the water probably prevents any actual back flow during this very short phase (c. 0.1 sec). (Hughes[89])

maintain the oxygenation of its blood. These and other ecological variations in patterns of irrigation in fishes are discussed by Hughes and Shelton.[89,93]

Counter-current flow in fish gills

The most effective uptake of oxygen from the irrigation stream results from a well-ordered flow of water over one side of the gill epithelium and an appropriately

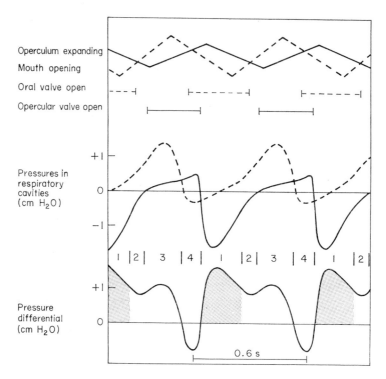

Operculum expanding

Mouth opening

Oral valve open

Opercular valve open

Pressures in
respiratory
cavities
(cm H₂O)

+1

0

−1

Pressure
differential
(cm H₂O)

+1

0

0.6 s

Fig. 7.3 Movements of the mouth and operculum with associated pressure changes in the buccal and opercular cavities in the trout. Broken lines represent the buccal side and continuous lines the opercular side of the system The upper record shows the operculum expansion and mouth opening cycles which are out of phase ; the second pair of lines indicate the relations of oral and opercular valve opening. The pressure changes are shown as separate records of actual observed pressures on either side of the gill resistance and below as the difference between the two sides ; shaded areas show the period when water flow is mainly due to the opercular suction pump. The figures above the pressure difference line refer to the phases illustrated by Fig. 7.2. The possibility of independent variation of the two pressures depends on the resistance to water flow afforded by the gill structure (see Fig. 7.4) and is essential to the elimination of intermittent flow. The short negative differential period may be further reduced and the opercular suction pump assume even greater importance in bottom-living forms such as the plaice. (After Hughes[89])

adjusted flow of blood in the *opposite direction* on the other. The principle of such a counter-current system, which is illustrated in Fig. 7.4, finds employment in a variety of other physiological fields in addition to gas exchange in the mammalian placenta (see Scholander[200]) and is well-known to engineers. Potentially, the recipient stream can come to equilibrium with the highest value in the donor stream instead of the two streams equilibrating at a mean value. Counter-

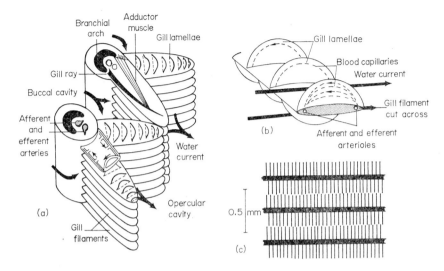

Fig. 7.4 The structure of the teleost gill and counter-current flow of blood and water. (a) Portions of two adjacent gill arches bearing double rows of filaments, which interlock at the tips—a passive posture due to the elasticity of the gill rays. Each filament bears rows of alternating lamellae on upper and lower faces in which the capillary blood flow runs counter to the flow of the water stream between the lamellae. (b) At higher magnification, part of a single filament with three lamellae above and below. (c) Diagrammatic representation of part of the seive-like arrangement provided by the filaments (3) and lamellae in the trench; the water flow is at right-angles to the page. (Hughes[88])

current involvement in the gas exchange of fishes was first appreciated by van Dam[36] and it undoubtedly contributes to the very high levels of utilization which characterize teleost gas exchange (p. 15). A proper adjustment of the two flow rates is also important and as Hughes has pointed out,[89] even with parallel flow a large volume of water moving rapidly past a small slowly moving stream of blood will yield a high degree of oxygenation of the blood but a low utilization; such an arrangement will supply the needed oxygen but at a high cost in irrigation metabolism.

Gill surface areas

Gill areas have been estimated in a number of groups. In a variety of molluscs, despite a diversity of gill forms, the values relative to body weight are remarkably constant and range from 7.1 cm²/g tissue weight in *Thais* (*Purpura*) *lapillus* to 9.3 in the cephalopod *Nautilus macromphalus* and 9.4 in *Patella vulgata*. Only in bivalves do the values rise appreciably, though not so much as might be expected, to 13.5 cm²/g in *Mytilus edulis* and *Cardium echinatum* (Pelseneer, quoted by Ghiretti[68]). These values may be compared with 10.9 cm²/g for the alveolar epithelium in man.

Studies of decapod crustacean gills in relation to habitat show some interesting surface area relations. Many crabs have adapted to a more-or-less terrestrial existence and there is a distinct tendency for the more thoroughly adapted species to have not only fewer gills but also smaller aggregate surface areas. Thus an active aquatic species, *Callinectes*, has 13.7 cm^2/g, the sluggish aquatic *Libinia dubia* 7.5, the intertidal *Uca pugilator* 6.3 and the land crab *Ocypode* 3.3.[71] A corresponding series of gill numbers goes 26, 18, 12.[166,167] Land crabs also tend to replace the original gills by alternative vascularized branchial tufts in the gill cavity. A reduction of the total gill area in land crabs is in keeping with the much higher oxygen content and easier ventilation in the new medium but presupposes that the branchial filaments are able to resist collapsing when no longer supported by water. The chitinous layer of the exoskeleton, which in an attenuated form is continuous over the gills, no doubt contributes to this desirable state of affairs. It is notable that land crabs do not seem to enjoy higher arterial pO_2s than their aquatic relatives (p. 106). In terrestrial isopods, such as *Ligia* and *Oniscus*, the gills serve well for air-breathing.

The fishes illustrate very well the common difficulty in using gills for aerial respiration. Here the unsupported gill lamellae collapse, a drastic reduction in effective exchange area occurs and asphyxiation commonly results. Some Gobies, including *Periophthalmus*, have structural support for the gills (by a coalescence of the lamellae) which renders air-breathing possible. Some other fishes, such as the carp, can survive for a while out of water by virtue of a marked bradycardia and tolerance of anaerobic metabolism analogous to the diving adaptations of some aquatic mammals (p. 161, 165).[89]

The areas of fish gills have been determined for a number of species and interesting correlations found. For average species with body weights around 100 g the area is about 4 cm^2/g, i.e. about twice the area of the external surface. In addition to a tendency for smaller and larger species to have larger and smaller relative areas respectively, there is a marked influence of activity. Thus, very active forms such as the mackerel (*Scomber*) and the herring (*Clupea*) have areas of about 10 cm^2/g, while sluggish bottom-feeders like the toadfish (*Opsanus*) have only about 2 cm^2/g. It seems very likely that individual species develop areas no larger than is necessary because this limits the area for salt and water flux and so minimizes the amount of osmotic work which must be performed.[3]

TRANSITION TO AIR-BREATHING

Transition to air-breathing in a number of groups has been stimulated by what Krogh has called 'emergency respiration'. Periodic withdrawal of water for intertidal animals produces a number of adaptations, many of them behavioural, but more protracted lack of oxygen in fresh water habitats, especially in tropical regions, has been the more important stimulus to the evolution of true air-breathing. There is a notable diversity of attempts to solve this problem among the fishes. While the aspiration of air bubbles over conventional gills may serve in some species such as *Hypopomus*, a tropical swamp fish from Paraguay,[28] many new structures are developed. Some of these, such as are found in *Pseudapocryptes*, *Gymnotus*, *Anabas*, *Clarias* and *Saccobranchus*, have been admirably reviewed by Krogh[128] and need not now be considered in detail. The common feature of these cases is the existence of enlarged, richly vascularized areas of buccal and pharyngeal epithelia, with or without rigid support. In some, regular ventilation movements are also found.

In yet other cases air is aspirated into more posterior parts of the alimentary canal such as the 'respiratory stomach' of *Plecostomus* into which air is swallowed, followed by regurgitation.[28] *Misgurnus*, the pond loach, goes even further; oxygen uptake from the swallowed air occurs in the mid-gut and hind-gut and the residual gas leaves via the anus.[98]

Recent work on the electric eel (*Electrophorus electricus*), a tropical obligate air-breather, has given an indication of the relatively high efficiency which can be achieved in uptake of oxygen from air via the buccal cavity.[49] The ventral and dorsal walls of the buccal cavity are extensively diverticulated and richly vascularized. At 26°C with a total oxygen uptake of 30 ml/kg/hr, 78% of oxygen is derived from the air. Most of the remaining 22% is exchanged through the scale-less skin, since the gills are atrophied and there are no irrigation movements. By contrast 81% of carbon dioxide exchange is via the skin. A similar striking imbalance of oxygen and carbon dioxide exchange is found in the lungfish *Protopterus* and in various amphibia (see p. 44).

The teleost swimbladder

None of these adaptations, evidently, could match the development of the separate pharyngeal gas bladder which has arisen independently a number of times and in different ways. The swimbladder, found in most teleosts, arises from and is connected via the pneumatic duct to the dorsal side of the alimentary canal. Although in modern forms principally a hydrostatic organ, it may in some physostomatous species, such as *Erythrinus*, have an accessory respiratory function. It would be difficult to establish with certainty whether the hydrostatic or the respiratory function is primitive. Early teleost evolution in potentially oxygen deficient fresh waters would point rather to an initial respiratory function, while later adaptation to a pelagic marine life in consistently oxygen-rich waters would swing the advantage towards hydrostasis which is certainly dominant in this group in recent times.

Although this hydrostatic function of the swimbladder is not strictly an aspect of respiration, a brief mention should be made of the method of filling the physoclystous type. There is not yet complete agreement about the mechanism but it does seem to depend in part upon a peculiar property of many fish haemoglobins. This is found in the reversible reduction of oxygen capacity caused by fall in pH—the Root effect. Since the gas gland in the swimbladder contains a highly developed *rete mirabile* system with the bends of its hairpin loops adjacent to the bladder lumen, it is supposed that local production of acidic meta-bolites (such as lactic acid) would turn out a substantial proportion of the bound oxygen reaching the loops, no matter what the prevailing pO_2. The liberated oxygen would be confined to the gland by counter-current exchange and a typical counter-current multiplication would occur, by virtue of the *rete* arrangement of the afferent and efferent capillaries. A pO_2 gradient from 0.2 to 200 atmospheres can occur across the gas gland wall and could in theory be created and sustained by exploiting the Root effect in conjunction with the *rete* system. This topic has been reviewed by Kuhn et al.[130] but later references are given by Wittenberg et al.[230]

A recent study of the primitive air-breathing fish *Amia calva* (the bowfin) shows that distribution of gas exchange between the gills and the air bladder varies with temperature and activity.[99] At 10°C the animal is relatively inactive and in air-saturated water the lungs provide only 8% of the oxygen and eliminate only 7% of the carbon dioxide. At 20°C the fish is much more active and there is a 5 times increase in oxygen uptake; then the lungs are responsible for 31% of oxygen and 23% of carbon dioxide exchange. Finally, at 30°C the metabolism is 6 times the initial level and 74% of oxygen is provided by the air bladder but most of the carbon dioxide is still eliminated via the gills. With falling pO_2 in the water there is a gradual increase in the rates of gill irrigation and of air bladder ventilation until at a pO_2 of 40 to 50 mm at 20°C ventilation sharply increased and irrigation declined. Changes in the blood gas tensions of systemic and air bladder vessels suggested a tendency for blood to bypass that gas exchange organ not primarily involved in oxygen uptake at any particular time.

The dipnoan lung

In vertebrate morphology the term 'lung' is usually reserved for structures which arise from the ventral side of the pharynx and necessarily remain connected to it, as in the Dipnoi (lungfishes) and in *Polypterus*. This structure, which even in its most primitive form is thought to have been bilobed, is the homologue of the lungs of tetrapods. As Krogh[128] has pointed out, such structures must satisfy certain well-defined conditions before they can be regarded as having respiratory function. These are (a) periodic ventilation; (b) lower pO_2 and higher pCO_2 in the expired air than in the atmosphere; (c) well-vascularized capillary epithelium and (d) frequently, but not invariably, an enlarged internal surface of epithelial ridges or pockets. It is not essential that the gas bladder be supplied with pure venous blood, though if it is the system is likely to be more efficient.

Hughes[89] has drawn attention to the diversity of vascular arrangements in accessory respiratory organs which seem on the whole to be dictated more by the anatomical derivation of the structures than by functional considerations. The success of the dipnoan type of lung development may have been due more than anything to the potentialities which existed for the evolution of efficient vascular arrangements. Thus, already in the lungfishes, separate pulmonary veins taking oxygenated blood through the incompletely divided heart and on to the first two branchial arches, effect a partial separation from venous blood going through the third and fourth arches and a special pulmonary artery to the lungs. The arrangements for separation of venous and arterial blood are further elaborated in amphibia and reptiles and reach perfection in the homoiotherms.

Although undoubtedly the dipnoan lung was at first an emergency development, in the African and S. American forms (*Protopterus* and *Lepidosiren* respectively) pulmonary respiration is now obligatory even in well-aerated water, the gills having been reduced to vestiges, with gill filaments surviving only on the fourth and fifth arches. These have perhaps a surviving osmo-regulatory salt-secretion function in addition to a slight but inadequate respiratory function.* The emergency situation, in the form of periodically dried out water courses and the need for aestivation, still remains but the emergency mechanism is now virtually exclusive. On the other hand the W. Australian *Neoceratodus* does not aestivate, is not an obligate air-breather and will die out of water.[100]

It is interesting that in *Lepidosiren paradoxa* the male forgoes any excursions to the surface during the period when it is mounting guard over the eggs in the nest. Associated with this habit is an enormous development of respiratory filaments on the pelvic fins; these start to appear just before mating and begin to atrophy at about 45 days after the eggs hatch. This coincides with the time when the larval gills begin to degenerate and the young fish begin to breathe air.[128]

The external gills of larval amphibia may also respond to changing availability of dissolved oxygen. In *Rana temporaria* and in *Salamandra* the gills are hypertrophied when dissolved oxygen is deficient and atrophied when the water is saturated or super-saturated.[63,128]

In a very interesting series of papers, Johansen and Lenfant have attempted to throw light on the physiological adaptations involved in the transition to air-breathing in lungfishes by experiments on *Neoceratodus*, *Lepidosiren* and *Protopterus* (see [101,139] for references). Both haemoglobin properties and respiratory performance indicate that *Neoceratodus* is essentially a gill-breather, able to use its lung as an auxiliary gas exchanger at times of lowered pO_2 in the water. On the other hand *Lepidosiren* and to an even greater extent *Protopterus* are thoroughly adapted to primary pulmonary uptake of oxygen, although both appear to rely still on the much reduced gills for carbon dioxide elimination. In *Protopterus* 89% of oxygen exchange but only 30% of carbon dioxide exchange takes place in the lung. Blood gas analyses from different parts of the circulatory system furnished physiological evidence of at least partial separation of oxygenated blood from systemic venous blood in a double circulation system previously postulated on anatomical grounds. It was suggested that the greater efficiency deriving from this advance enables lungfishes to survive with bloods of rather

---

* The author found to his cost, when trying to obtain living *Protopterus* in Uganda, that the fishermen of the L. Kyoga region are increasingly giving up the traditional tall, conical basket traps which when set in shallow water rise above the surface and permit the lungfish access to the air. When caught on hooks instead the fish frequently drown before the lines are hauled.

lower oxygen capacity (5–8 vols %) than are found in air-breathing teleosts (12–18 vols %). Some other features of this work are referred to later (p. 129). Lenfant and Johansen[138] also examined the air-breathing transition in a series of amphibia showing increasing dependence on the lungs. *Necturus maculosus* is a neotenic form, fully aquatic with poor lungs but well-developed external gills. *Amphiuma tridactylum* is an aquatic form devoid of gills but with a well-developed lung. *Rana catesbeiana* is largely terrestrial with well-developed lungs. Most of the important respiratory pigment properties and the blood gas parameters were found to reflect the progressively increased dependence on pulmonary gas exchange through this series (see also p. 58).

LUNGS

Most air-breathing animals, whose metabolic needs cannot be met by cutaneous respiration, have specialized invaginated epithelia for gas exchange. Although these are found in many different forms, they may all be referred to as lungs. Invaginated respiratory organs are less subject than aerial gills to water loss by evaporation from their necessarily moist epithelia because of the possibility of limiting and regulating the amount of air to which they are exposed; they also enjoy a measure of protection not possible, at least for external gills. On the other hand, since the great majority of lungs which animals have developed do not lend themselves to a through-flow ventilation, carbon dioxide partial pressure in the pulmonary gas rises to much higher levels than the virtually ambient level found in the stream over a well-irrigated gill. This leads to a new possibility for respiratory regulation (p. 148). The relatively high pulmonary pCO_2 encourages elimination via the general body surface, directly into the air (or water) which is practically CO_2-free, whenever the nature of the integument permits, as we have seen already in terrestrial amphibia (p. 44) in lung-fishes (p. 55) and in other air-breathing fishes (p. 53, 54).

Diffusion lungs

In the simplest lung systems the maintenance of the optimum pulmonary gas mixture depends on diffusion alone but since diffusion even in gases has its limitations this can only serve for relatively small or inactive animals. The largest animals depending on diffusion lungs are probably the African pulmonate snails, *Achatina* and *Bulinus*, with volumes up to 500 ml.[128]

Diffusion lungs seem to be the rule in pulmonate gastropods, whether aquatic or terrestrial. Ghiretti[68] quotes some work which suggests that active ventilation movements occur in *Helix pomatia*. It is apparent that on closure of the pneumostome in this species, relaxation of the muscles in the arched mantle floor results in a gradual increase of pulmonary pressure which may well facilitate diffusion of oxygen into the pulmonary capillary system. When the pneumostome reopens, the pressure falls to normal and the mantle floor contracts to increase the volume again. These movements will certainly help to 'top-up' the lung with fresh air but in the absence of good evidence for rhythmic volume change while the pneumostome is open, the term ventilation is hardly justified. Krogh[128] discusses the evidence on this point in some detail and denies any respiratory significance for these movements. Pulmonary oxygen uptake is supplementary to cutaneous exchange especially in aquatic pulmonates and in these forms the lung is probably quite insignificant for carbon dioxide elimination (p. 119). The relative lung area in shelled pulmonates seems to be comparable with that of mammals, e.g. 8.3 cm^2/g tissue weight in *Helix pomatia* against 10.9 in man but in the naked slugs it is much lower, about 0.7 cm^2/g in *Arion*,[128] presumably reflecting a greater ease of cutaneous exchange.

The arachnids make use of diffusion lungs of a rather elaborate kind. These are well exemplified by the 'book lungs' of spiders in which the pulmonary cavities, protected by spiracles, are completely subdivided by many parallel lamellae (resembling the pages of a book) perfused with haemolymph. Scorpions also have segmentally arranged lungs of essentially the same type. The interstices and tubular extensions of the subdivided pulmonary cavities in these and similar devices (e.g. in some isopods and in myriopods) are often called 'tracheae'. However, it must be realized that the usual function of these air spaces is oxygenation of the haemolymph. The distinction between diffusion lung and tracheal system is sometimes difficult to draw in this phylum.

Some authors have described movements of supposed respiratory significance in many kinds of diffusion lung but Krogh[128] has asserted that wherever the dimensions are adequately known, diffusion is calculably adequate to account for the observed exchanges.

Ventilation lungs

The energetic vertebrates alone have developed air-breathing lungs with mechanisms for regular ventilation. Although such a system evidently makes large size with a high metabolic rate possible, it does not (any more than in the diffusion lung) permit the full exploitation of the consistently high pO$_2$ of the medium. The tidal ventilation mechanism ensures a marked dilution of inspired air with residual air and alveolar pO$_2$ does not normally exceed 105 mm. This limitation is only partially overcome in birds with the tendency towards a through-flow system (p. 67). However, the appropriate adjustment of the loading tension of the haemoglobin (p. 57) and the relatively low cost of ventilation in air (p. 16) combine with the superior blood/gas equilibration conditions in the lung to compensate for the loss of at about one-third of the potential pO$_2$ gradient.

The factors governing pulmonary function in man have been exhaustively studied and described in many standard texts. Conditions in other groups are much less understood. For the present it is sufficient to note a few comparative aspects.

The lungs of amphibia are quite simple and even in the more complex examples (e.g. *Rana*) have modest areas in relation to body weight. Increasing complexity of structure leads progressively to larger relative surface areas and shorter diffusion pathways in reptiles and mammals. The trend which is illustrated in Fig. 7.5 represents not only increasing metabolic rate but also decreasing capacity for cutaneous exchange. Only in amniotes can a true distinction be made between the gas exchange alveoli and the dead-space air passages of trachea and bronchial system. The functional extent of these developments can be indicated by comparison of some pulmonary parameters for frog and man (Table 7.1).

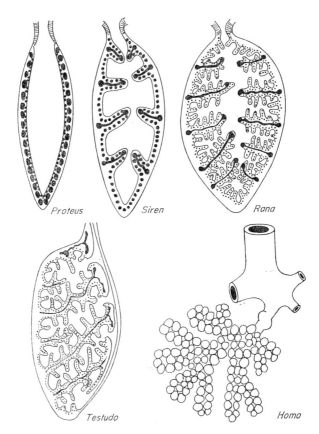

Fig. 7.5 Diagrammatic representation of the structure of the lungs in amphibians (*Proteus, Siren* and *Rana*), reptiles (*Testudo*) and mammals (*Homo*). In the last example only a single alveolar unit opening from a final bronchus is shown. In amphibian lungs the whole inner surface is lined by capillaries (the smaller black spots) and is used in gas exchange. In the reptilian lung there is the beginning of a separation of airways or bronchi from the alveoli, which reaches its peak in mammals. Note that the individual mammalian alveoli are not of uniform size. The mammalian capillaries are not shown; they form a network over the outside of the alveoli. (Redrawn from Krogh[128])

Table 7.1 Pulmonary area and volume relationships in frog, pigeon and man. All values are approximate; the smaller lung area for man is an estimate of alveolar surface in contact with capillaries (diffusion area); for the pigeon, the larger lung volume includes air-sacs and the area/volume ratio is a calculated value for the crow. (From Krogh[122,128] (frog); Comroe[32] (man) and Sturkie[207] (birds))

	Lung vol. (ml)	Lung area (cm²)	Lung area / lung vol. (cm²/ml)	Lung area / body wt. (cm²/g)	Tidal vol. (ml)	Tidal vol. as % total lung vol.
Frog	5	100	20	8.4	—	—
Man	3000	900 000 (700 000)	300	11	450	15
Pigeon	8–70	160	(20)	0.5	5	62–7

The comparative structure of amphibian and reptilian lungs has recently been intensively studied by Tenney and Tenney.[208]

Amphibian lungs

Much uncertainty, not usually apparent in the simpler textbook accounts, has surrounded the ventilation mechanism of the amphibian lung. For the bullfrog *Rana catesbeiana*, at least, the matter has been much clarified in a recent sophisticated and painstaking investigation by de Jongh and Gans.[111] The basic features of their findings, which related pressure changes and muscle activities, are represented in Fig. 7.6.

With the glottis tightly closed, there is a background of bucco-pharyngeal movements at a frequency of 50 to 100 cycles per minute which pump air in and out of the open nostrils; compression is due to intermandibular, inter- and geniohyoid muscles, while expansion is due to relaxation of these muscles and the buccal floor falling under its own weight. The pressure change has an amplitude of about 0.5 cm H_2O equally above and below atmospheric; hence these are called 'oscillatory cycles'.

Periodically a more complex 'ventilation cycle' starts with a contraction of the sternohyoid muscle which causes a more pronounced lowering of the buccal floor and buccal pressure (phase 1). With buccal pressure at its minimum, the glottis opens; air previously under considerable pressure leaves the lungs, due to equalization of the pulmonary and buccal pressures and elastic contraction of the lungs, and the excess escapes through the nostrils (phase 2). Purely passive exhalation is therefore immediately preceded by maximal filling of the buccal cavity with fresh air. A third phase of variable prominence sees a slight further escape of air and fall in pressure in the lungs; due to the resistance to flow through the nostrils, buccal pressure remains above atmospheric pressure but levels off. Then for the first and only time the nostrils close, the buccal floor is strongly contracted (the petro- and omohyoid muscles being involved this time) and a

c

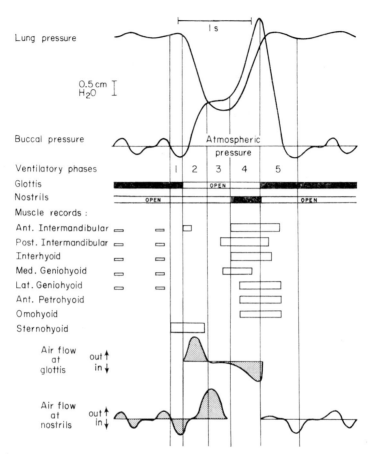

Fig. 7.6 Schematic representation of some events during oscillatory and ventilatory cycles in *Rana catesbeiana*. The record begins and ends with an oscillatory cycle; pulmonary pressure changes during these cycles (glottis closed) are indirectly due to posture changes in the buccal region. The time and pressure magnitudes as indicated by the scales are characteristic but not invariable. Pressure changes, opening and closing of glottis and nostrils and muscular contractions as observed; air flow at glottis and nostrils estimated from consideration of pressure differentials, state of the valves and other characteristics of the system. Movements of the flanks are omitted from the record (inward during phase 2 and outward during phase 4); these are thought to be a passive consequence of the changes in lung volume as there is no evidence of an active role. Note the specialized role of the sternohyoid and of the petro- and omohyoid muscles in expanding and contracting respectively the posterior buccal cavity. (Redrawn with some simplification from de Jongh and Gans[111])

sharp rise in buccal pressure causes reinflation of the lung (phase 4). The final phase begins with simultaneous closing of the glottis, reopening of the nostrils and a drop in buccal pressure; the muscles which lift the buccal floor are relaxed so that it again falls under gravity and the phase and cycle end with sub-atmospheric pressure sucking air into the buccal cavity and leading into the next sequence of oscillatory cycles.

A longer-term 'inflation cycle' was also described. For a period each ventilation cycle is followed by several oscillatory cycles and the peak pressure (end of phase 4) remains constant. This is followed by a period with fewer interspersed oscillatory cycles and a progressive increase in the peak pressure from one ventilatory cycle to the next until a 200 to 300% increase in the maximum pressure is obtained. Thereafter 5 to 15 oscillatory cycles follow without ventilation. Finally this apneic period is followed by a sequence of closely approximated ventilatory cycles with progressively diminished peak pressures. These long-term cycles take up to 2 minutes at 25°C.

Several pieces of evidence suggest that the air expired through the glottis impinges in a stream directly on the internal nares during phase 2 and thus escapes with minimal mixing with the freshly inhaled air (phase 1) which mainly lies in a deep cavity in the posterior buccal floor (created by contraction of the sternohyoid muscles). This awaits inspiration in phase 4 with the contraction of the petro- and omohyoid muscles. However, a considerable amount of expired air remains in the buccal cavity after inspiration is complete and the function of the oscillatory cycles is seen as flushing this out prior to the next ventilatory cycle and not related to buccal gas exchange.

That the system does attain high levels of pulmonary pO_2 is indicated by the high arterial pO_2 (95 mm) and low oxygen affinity of the haemoglobin ($p_{50} = 39$ mm) found in *R. catesbeiana* by Lenfant and Johansen.[138] In this respect and in this species, at least, the buccal-force pump seems to do as well as the costal suction-pump of mammals. In *R. esculenta* p_{50} is 27 mm, as in man.

Foxon[63] has suggested that the buccal force-pump of modern amphibia is a secondary feature correlated with loss of the ribs. However, a recent study by McMahon[154] has revealed an essentially similar mechanism for lung ventilation in *Protopterus*. The similarity includes the curious feature of inhalation into the buccal cavity before expiration from the lung but the open mouth allows the passage of air rather than the nostrils. Furthermore, McMahon has shown that ventilation in this lungfish is effected by minor modifications of a sequence of three normal gill irrigation cycles. These irrigation cycles in turn are basically the same as those responsible for the dual-pumping mechanism of teleosts and elasmobranchs, including buccal compression and expansion phases. In lungfish ventilation the first compression empties the buccal cavity of water and the first expansion (with the mouth out of water) encompasses the requisite amount of air, followed by opening of the glottis and passive expiration. The second compression (both the mouth and opercular flap now closed) serves to inflate the lung. Following this the fish sinks below the surface so that the second expansion fills the buccal cavity with water and the third compression uses this to displace any residual air out of the buccal and opercular cavities via the oper-culum. Sometimes an additional cycle is interpolated for additional inhalation and inspiration without expiration.

McMahon develops the interesting hypothesis that a basically similar buccal-opercular branchial pumping mechanism is found in all fishes and that when the exigencies of the aquatic habitat put a premium on auxiliary or alternative aerial respiration, the machinery was readily adapted both in lungfishes and amphibia for purposes of lung ventilation.

Reptilian lungs

Nowhere among the lungfishes or amphibia is there involvement of the ribs in ventilation, a feature which seems to await the radically new costal suction-pump development of the reptiles. This is usually held to be more efficient than the buccal force-pump but the work on *Rana catesbeiana* discussed above seems to argue otherwise.

The ventilation of typical reptilian lungs has not been the subject of such care-ful and sophisticated analysis as that of *Rana* and *Protopterus* but a triphasic pattern of respiratory movements has been described for the lizard *Lacerta*.[88] With the glottis open, contraction of abdominal muscles and of the smooth muscles of the lungs themselves produces an expiration. Inspiration follows immediately by active expansion of the rib cage (contraction of intercostal muscles), the lungs reaching a larger volume than immediately preceding the expiration. The glottis then closes with the lung fully inflated at atmospheric pressure. Then follows a partial 'expiratory' movement of a passive nature due to movement of the abdominal viscera; since this occurs with the glottis closed the pressure of the pulmonary air rises slightly and is sustained above atmos-pheric. There follows a definite pause before the glottis opens and the next proper expiration occurs. The costal suction-pump facilitates inspiration of really fresh air, though it is still diluted by the residual air.

Although the nostrils are provided with sphincters and bucco-pharyngeal movements are often seen during the pauses, they are not thought to have a respiratory significance in most forms; they are probably olfactory. In some aquatic turtles, however, this bucco-pharyngeal ventilation may serve for a measure of aquatic respiration while submerged and so help to eke out the pulmonary oxygen 'store'.[89] Small air sacs are found in communication with the lungs in some lizards such as *Chamaeleo*. Their function is unknown but they seem to foreshadow the very extensive air sac development of birds.

The costal pump mechanism has of necessity been modified in those chelo-nians which are enclosed within a rigid box. In *Testudo graeca* a thorough analysis shows that the triphasic pattern with a final recompression phase after closure of the glottis is still present. The active changes in lung volume are achieved by pressures transmitted through the viscera. The transverse abdominal and the oblique abdominal muscles respectively pull in or pull out the tissues which seal the posterior shell aperture while the pectoralis and seratus major muscles respectively cause inward or outward movements of the pectoral girdle and forelimbs.[67]

Mammalian lungs

Moving on to the mammals, we find again that improved pulmonary performance is based on an enormous development of lung structure allied to still further refinement of the ventilation mechanism.* The costal pump is in this case provided with two sets of antagonistic intercostal muscles, the external intercostals producing an active enlargement of the rib cage for inspiration. In the resting state, expiration is largely due to the elasticity of the lung itself but contraction of the internal intercostals is involved when high ventilation volumes are required. In addition, the development of the muscular diaphragm enables the lungs to be enclosed in pleural cavities which are quite separate from the other body cavities. The contraction of this partition, which is convex anteriorly, results in an enlargement of the pleural cavities sufficient to account for almost all the 500 ml of resting inspiration (in man). The costal and diaphragmic pumps are therefore to a large extent alternatives and are used in differing degrees. The orientation of the ribs in human infants makes costal pumping inefficient, so diaphragm pumping is relied upon. Adult females use the costal muscles to a greater extent than males, while in quadrupedal and aquatic mammals the diaphragm is most important.

The activities of these two mechanisms for suction-pumping cause a simple cycle of pressure changes in the pleural cavities ranging from about 4 to 9 mm below atmospheric. Corresponding changes within the lungs are substantially damped by consequential air movements. Minimal intrapulmonic pressure (early inspiration) is about 2 mm below and maximal pressure (early expiration) about 2.5 mm above atmospheric pressure. The pressure at end-inspiration is atmospheric since in contrast to the situation in amphibia and reptiles, there is no closure of the glottis. Also the rhythm of inspiration/expiration is normally uninterrupted by significant pauses.

Lung structure in mammals is characterized by the most extensive development of air-passages which are quite separate from the gas exchange sites in the alveoli. The result is an extensive dead-space, of about 140 ml in man, so that about 28% of the 500 ml inspired air in the resting state (tidal volume) fails to reach the region of gas exchange. However, increased oxygen demand can greatly increase the volume of inspired air up to about 3600 ml in healthy young males. Depth of expiration may also increase so that a maximal tidal volume (vital capacity) of 4800 ml may be reached and the anatomic dead-space then becomes relatively insignificant. Even at the extreme limit of expiration there remains a residual volume of about 1200 ml exclusive of dead-space. The residual used air must always be mixed with the inspired air, so lowering the alveolar composition markedly below the 150 mm pO_2 which the water-saturated inspired air has in

* The following account is largely based on the texts of Comroe[32] and Comroe et al.[33]

the trachea and which would obtain in the alveoli if the lung were capable of being completely emptied. The minimal residual volume constitutes about 20% and the resting residual volume (functional residual capacity) about 40% of the total lung capacity of 6000 ml.

The rate at which oxygen can be absorbed into the pulmonary circulation depends on the stabilization of the alveolar pO_2 and this in turn depends more on the rate and amount of alveolar ventilation than on total lung volume or on actual residual volume. In fact the residual air plays an important part in buffering alveolar pO_2 against the changes which occur with each inspiration/expiration cycle. The observed changes range from about 98 to 101 mm pO_2 with a mean of about 99.7 mm, while for carbon dioxide the range is from 38 to 40.7 mm with a mean of about 39.2 mm.

The structure of the mammalian lung is too complex to be represented in Fig. 7.5 in a comparable manner to the simpler forms. Instead a single bronchial twig and its alveoli are shown. Each human lung contains about 3 to 3.5 $\times 10^8$ alveoli which individually have diameters ranging from 75 to 300 μm. The total alveolar surface is about 90 m^2 and the diffusion area actually in contact with blood capillary walls is about 70 m^2. The combined thickness of alveolar epithelium and capillary endothelium is less than 0.1 μm. On the vascular side, although the capillaries have a diameter of only 7 to 10 μm, the total resistance to flow is so low that at rest a difference in blood pressure from 25/8 to 5 mm can drive blood through the system at 5 to 10 l/min. In maximal exercise this rate can rise to 30 to 40 l/min.

Efficient gas exchange requires a precise balancing of the alveolar ventilation against capillary circulation rate at all levels of oxygen demand and in those homoiotherms which regulate temperature largely by pulmonary-water evaporation, the nature of the ventilation must be adjusted at the same time to regulate water loss. Thus shallow breathing will result in evaporation from the dead-space surfaces without the danger of hyperventilation of the alveoli.

The complexity of the air passages and the number of the alveoli, compared with the reptilian condition, make for considerable problems in achieving uniformity of ventilation. Likewise, uniformity of blood flow through such an extensive capillary bed is important and presents greater problems in the most advanced lungs. Uneven ventilation will have adverse effects on oxygen uptake because reduced percentage saturation of blood exposed to hypoventilated alveoli cannot be compensated by correspondingly increased saturation of blood exposed to hyperventilated alveoli. This is a consequence of the changing slope of the upper-end of the dissociation curve on which the arterial point falls when the oxygen affinity of the haemoglobin is well-adapted (Fig. 9.1, p. 98). Even in normal lungs a slight lack of uniformity of ventilation occurs and arterial saturation at 97.1% falls short of the 'ideal' value of 97.4%. The deficiency is much greater as result of a number of pathological factors which further diminish the uniformity of ventilation and of circulation.

Avian lungs

The lungs of birds with their remarkable air sac system are built on a different pattern from those of other vertebrates and are ventilated in a distinctive manner. There are a number of excellent summaries of the morphology and ventilation mechanism[89,128,193,207] but a brief account will help to highlight the differences. The principal features are represented in Fig. 7.7.

The trachea divides into two primary bronchi as usual but each of these continues right through the lung as a broad mesobronchus which terminates in a cluster of up to sixteen posterior secondary bronchi and also opens into the largest abdominal air sac and the thoracic air sac. Each posterior secondary bronchus communicates with numerous tertiary bronchi or parabronchi. The bulk of the lung is made up of a relatively solid, densely packed mass of these parabronchi which arborize and freely anastomose in a system of through-conducting tubes. The packing is facilitated by the hexagonal section of the individual tubes, each of which is about 1 mm across and with a bore of about 0.5 mm. Opening from the lumen and penetrating into the wall are very large numbers of fine, arborizing, blind-ending tubes.* It is in these air capillaries, with diameters up to 10 μm, that the gas exchange takes place, since they are ultimately separated from the blood in the parabronchial wall only by the endothelium of the pulmonary capillaries. The bronchial circuit is completed by fusion of the parabronchi until they open into four anterior secondary bronchi, which in turn open into the anterior region of the mesobronchus. The anterior air sacs (cervical, inter-clavicular and anterior thoracic) also open into the anterior secondary bronchi. One further feature (not mentioned by Hughes[89] or Salt and Zeuthen[193]) possibly of great functional importance, is an arrangement of recurrent bronchi which arise from the proximal ends of the air sacs, especially of the abdominal and posterior thoracics. These recurrent bronchi were thought to anastomose freely with the parabronchial system and form a potential route to and/or from the air sacs other than via the mesobronchus. Akester[1] recognizes the recurrent bronchi in development but since they appear like parabronchi, doubts they have any special significance in the adult.

There still is no complete agreement about the details of the ventilation of this complex system. Basically, a costal suction-pump produces inspiration by enlargement of the lungs (which are firmly adherent to the ribs but relatively inelastic compared with other vertebrate lungs) and more important, by enlargement of the air sacs. Expiration is partly due to relaxation of the external intercostals, contraction of the internal intercostals and dropping of the sternum. The abdominal muscles and diaphragm seem to be unimportant but in flight the rhythmic raising and lowering of the sternum by the flight muscles has an important ventilation role.

The air pathway within the system is not certainly established but a number of

---

* Krogh[128] says that the air capillaries of different parabronchi anastomose with one another but this is probably true of strong fliers only.[193]

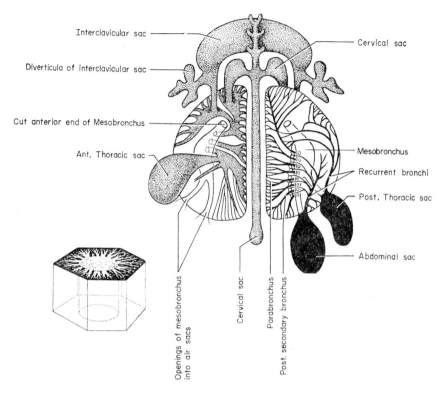

Fig. 7.7 Diagrammatic representation of the lungs and air sacs of a bird. Left, ventral view; right, dorsal view. The trachea and primary bronchi are omitted. In representing the air sacs the shapes have been simplified and the relative sizes changed (see Table 7.2). Inspiratory sacs black; expiratory sacs stippled. Only the superficial parts of the para-bronchial systems are shown; in fact the whole thickness of the lung is occupied by these ramifications. Inset is a section of a single parabronchus showing branching of the air capillaries from the central lumen. (After Portmann)[170]

hypotheses can be reduced to two basic alternatives. The first (mainly due to Hazelhoff[79]) involves an expiratory flow through the parabronchi which is in one direction, namely from the posterior air sacs via both the well-developed recurrent bronchi and the posterior secondary bronchi. The expired air leaves the parabronchi via the anterior secondary bronchi and the anterior end of the mesobronchus. Expiration also tends to empty the anterior sacs.

In this scheme inspiration is characterized by three features: (a) access of fresh air to the posterior sacs directly via the mesobronchus; (b) topping-up of the anterior sacs with used air from the parabronchi via the anterior secondary bronchi; (c) refilling of the parabronchi with fresh air via the posterior secondary bronchi. Thus there would be a through-flow in the one direction only. These ideas accord with a number of observed features including the consistently lower pO_2 and higher pCO_2 in the anterior sacs compared with the posterior sacs (Table 7.2). It is not easy to see how this mechanism would operate without a well-developed arrangement of valves (which have never been seen) but there is a 'guiding dam' at the posterior end of the mesobronchus which might help.

The second scheme (see Salt and Zeuthen[193]) involves movement of part of the air flow through the parabronchi in one direction at inspiration and in the reverse direction at expiration. The remaining air flow would be to and from the posterior air sacs via the mesobronchus. The relative total cross-sectional areas and resistances of the mesobronchus and the parabronchial system are such that there would always be a reasonable parabronchial flow, even without valves and this is calculated at 29–48% of the air reaching the posterior air sacs during inspiration and 38–67% of the air leaving during expiration. Whichever system operates, oxygen and carbon dioxide must diffuse a mean distance of about 0.3 to 0.4 mm from the parabronchial lumen to the air capillaries. Hazelhoff[69] calculated that such a diffusion situation could supply a total of about 2 l of oxygen per minute in the crow.

The combined ventilation of air sacs and lungs enables the bird to achieve exceptionally high rates of oxygen uptake with a relatively very small area for actual gas exchange. This is apparent from a comparison of the lung area relative to lung volume or body weight in pigeon and man (Table 7.1).

Most authors agree that this elaborate system is highly adaptive and more efficient than the simple tidal ventilation of other vertebrate lungs. Yet it is not entirely clear where the advantages lie. Through-flow (either uni-directional or bi-directional) in the parabronchi could result in a higher alveolar (air capillary) pO_2 than is possible in a tidal system. This has not been directly determined and the pO_2 of deep expired air may not be a reliable indirect indication as it is in a tidal system. Values for partial pressures in expired air and in the various air sacs are given in Table 7.2. If the parabronchi receive 'fresh' air from the posterior sacs or direct from the mesobronchus and if the anterior sacs contain largely vitiated air, the parabronchial pO_2 will no doubt be substantially higher than the 100 mm alveolar pO_2 found in man. Diffusion into the air capillaries is probably no more of a problem than it is from the mouth of a normal alveolus with a diameter of 75 to 300 μm. Such a superior 'alveolar' pO_2 would be consistent with the generally lower oxygen affinity of bird haemoglobins (p. 100). The system may also promote greater utilization, since the expired air can contain as little as 14.5 vols% oxygen in duck and pigeon and 13.5 vols% in chicken compared with 16.4 vols% in man.[207]

Krogh[128] has drawn attention to the capacity of the total system to provide a finely regulated means of evaporative temperature regulation but this is not an adequate *raison d'être*.[193] Sturkie[207] points out that reasonable respiratory exchange can occur after destruction of all the air sacs and discusses a number of fanciful alternative roles which have been suggested for the air sacs *per se*. It seems likely that the full adaptive significance of the system will be related to

C 2

Table 7.2 Volumes and composition of the contents of the air sacs and of the expired air in the duck. Volumes (in ml) are the total for the pairs of sacs except for the interclavicular which is unpaired .(Sturkie)[207]

	Volume	% O_2	% CO_2
Interclavicular	53	13.1–14.2	6.0–5.6
Anterior thoracic	24	14.9	5.1
Posterior thoracic	57	17.7	2.7
Abdominal	145	17.2–18.1*	2.7–2.5
Expired air	38	14.3–15.8	5.1–3.0

* The maximum air sac % O^2 corresponds to 127 mm pO^2 at a body temperature of 41 °C. (cf. alveolar pO_2 of 100 mm in man).

flight and therefore its revelation will depend on mastering the difficulties of measuring normal respiratory parameters on the wing.

Pulmonary surfactants

The development of the alveolar ventilation lung in the vertebrates introduced a new physical factor into respiratory function—surface tension. A problem is posed by the existence of a gas/fluid interface lining each alveolus. This was brought to light only in 1929, by the discovery that the pressure required to inflate to a given volume a liquid-filled lung, in which there is no interfacial surface tension, is less than half that required to inflate it to the same volume when filled with gas. It was then clear that the 'elasticity' of the lung is dependent on more than the elastic fibres within the tissues which would function equally well in liquid-filled or gas-filled lungs.

Without going into surface tension theory, it can be stated that if the liquid at the interface were simply plasma, having a surface tension of 50 dynes/cm, the pressure needed to inflate the lung would be 20000 dynes/cm²—equivalent to about 20 cm H_2O. Such a pressure is required for maximal artificial inflation but is 5 to 10 times greater than that needed for artificial inflation to normal volume. Surface tension in the lung proves to be high when fully inflated but low when normally inflated and very low when deflated. There must be, therefore, some surface active material (surfactant) present in the interfacial liquid which lowers the surface tension when the film is contracted and raises it when expanded.

Furthermore, 'soap-bubble' physics indicates that the pressure inside a static bubble is inversely proportional to its radius. If the alveoli behaved like soap-bubbles, one would therefore expect that different pressures would occur inside the different sized alveoli of the expanded lung. This is clearly not possible because of the continuity of the air passages. The only alternative would be for the smaller alveoli to empty themselves into the larger, with the result that the lung would consist partly of collapsed and partly of over-inflated alveoli. This is certainly not true of healthy lungs. The fluid lining the alveoli must have rather

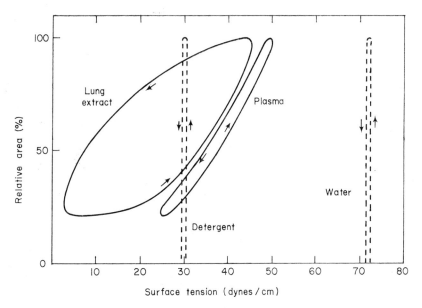

Fig. 7.8 Variation of surface tension during cycles of compression and expansion of liquid films. Films of water or detergent have the same tension whatever the area, though tension in a detergent film may be less than half that in water. Blood plasma films have higher tensions when expanded than when compressed. A film of lung extract not only shows this area/tension dependence but also for a given area there is a markedly higher tension in a film which is tending to expand than in one which is tending to contract. Pulmonary surfactants therefore have a powerful stabilizing effect on the area (and volume) of alveoli of different sizes. (After Comroe)[32]

special surface action properties and this is made clear by consideration of Fig. 7.8.

Fluid extracts from the lung do have the properties required to explain the observed behaviour. The surfactant is a complex lipoprotein based on dipalmitoyl lecithin. The complete absence of this material from the lining fluid may lead to total collapse of the alveoli on expiration and this is a feature of the congestive collapse of the lungs from a variety of causes. Absence or inactivation of the surfactant is also found in the respiratory distress syndrome of the newborn.

A simple but fuller account of the theory of surfactants is given in the textbook by Comroe.[32] Pattle has reviewed this field[164] and has given a summary of the comparative picture throughout the vertebrates.[165] Pulmonary surfactants have been found in the lungs of *Protopterus*, *Lepidosteus* the garpike (but not in teleost swimbladders), *Rana*, *Xenopus* and various reptiles and birds as well as in mammals. The only negative finding is among the urodeles—*Triton vulgaris* is the only one so far examined. The lungs of birds and mammals contain considerable reserves of surfactant but this appears not to be the case in the poikilotherms.

Water lungs

Invaginated surfaces are occasionally used for gas exchange in aquatic animals. In this category might be included the bucco-pharyngeal irrigation of some aquatic turtles (*Amyda* and *Aspidonotus*) already mentioned (p. 62). It is said that in an Amazon turtle (*Podocnemys*) rhythmic irrigation of the well-developed cloacal bursae can account for up to 90% of the oxygen uptake under certain conditions (reported by Steen,[247] p. 132). This kind of arrangement has also been demonstrated as having respiratory significance in a very few invertebrates.

Probably the best developed example is found in the respiratory trees of many holothurians. These paired structures which lie in the extensive perivisceral coelom, are hollow outgrowths of the cloaca in the form of a long central rhachis and very numerous arborizing side branches. Expiration is effected by contraction of the body wall muscles and of the respiratory trees themselves and inspiration is by a pumping action of the cloaca. Gas exchange takes place between the inspired sea-water and the coelomic fluid through the thin walls of the fine branches of the tree. When cloacal irrigation is prevented, oxygen uptake falls by about 50%. Evidently the tentacles, tube-feet and general body surface retain a substantial gas exchange function as in other echinoderms.[50] Within the perivisceral coelom of holothurians, cells containing haemoglobin are often found; they are theoretically more likely to have a storage function than a transport function (p. 140), although this matter has not been investigated.

In the gephyrean worm *Urechis caupo* the whole of the thin-walled hind gut constitutes a respiratory organ and the pumping action of the cloaca results in a regular rhythmic irrigation with sea-water. Here gas exchange between the gut water and the coelomic fluid is facilitated by the stirring action of peristaltic waves in the gut wall itself. Again the coelomic fluid contains erythrocytes and the question of storage or transport function is discussed in detail later (p. 140).

Claims for the respiratory significance of gut irrigation have been made for a number of annelids but Krogh[128] concludes that satisfactory evidence is lacking and that adequate branchial and cutaneous exchange occurs in all these cases.

Finally, mention must be made of the possibility that the primarily air-breathing lung of aquatic pulmonate snails may on occasions be used as a water lung. It is known that in some forms, such as *Lymnaea pereger* and *Physa fontinalis* which live remote from the shore line, the lung may be water-filled throughout life.[94] However, it has not been demonstrated that in these conditions any sort of irrigation of the lung occurs. There is no good evidence of active ventilation when these organs are used for air-breathing (pp. 57 and 116).

TRACHEAL RESPIRATION

Morphology and ventilation

Apart from some general cutaneous exchange in small aquatic forms, none of the foregoing descriptions of respiratory organs can be applied to insects. In this group respiratory gas exchange, like various other physiological functions (osmoregulation and excretion, sensory perception, etc.) involves organs which are unique. From the standpoint of our overall comparative picture of respiration, the cardinal distinction is the virtual exclusion of the insect vascular system from any part in the transport of respiratory gases. Instead these highly original animals have developed a method in which gas exchange and transport are combined within a single anatomic entity, the tracheal system.

Since, therefore, consideration of respiratory organs does not lead on to questions of the properties of the blood as a gas transport medium and since there are a number of excellent recent accounts of tracheal respiration (e.g. by Wigglesworth[226] and Miller[156]), our treatment of this topic will be brief and confined to physiological essentials. Tracheal systems also subserve a number of non-respiratory functions which have been listed and briefly described by Miller.[156]

Between the insect tracheal system proper and the diffusion lungs of the other terrestrial arthropods (p. 57) there is an area in which a firm line of distinction is difficult to draw. In all but the more primitive spiders, lung books are supplemented by 'tracheae' but since these seem to serve for oxygenating the haemolymph, they should be regarded as lungs. In the Onycophora, Solifugae, Phalangidae, some Acarina and Myriapoda, the larger part of the tracheal system appears to be engaged in conducting oxygen directly to the tissues. In the Insecta, a few larval forms (*Hypoderma* and Tipulidae) have some tracheoles lying free in the haemolymph but their respiratory significance is obscure.[128]

The by-passing of the vascular system is made possible by the extraordinarily far-reaching ramifications of the tubular tracheae and tracheoles, which permit the direct diffusion of gaseous oxygen to and carbon dioxide from the respiring cells (Fig. 7.9). Commonly, the outer-end of the system is guarded by a spiracular mechanism, permitting contact with the atmosphere to be regulated with some precision in the interests of water conservation. The tracheae have an outer epithelium continuous with the epidermis and an inner layer continuous with the cuticle. This cuticular lining is usually provided with annular or spiral thickenings (taenidia) to prevent occlusion of the lumen. The tracheoles, which spring in considerable numbers from the proximal end of each ultimate tracheal branch, consist of minute intracellular tubes. Electron microscope studies show that the spiral thickening is still present. Unlike tracheae, tracheoles are not shed with the moult. Gas exchange, as in the more highly developed alveolar lungs, is confined to these microscopic extremities of the system in contact with the tissues and even with individual cells.

The spiracles, which are arranged in bilaterally symmetrical pairs, are, except

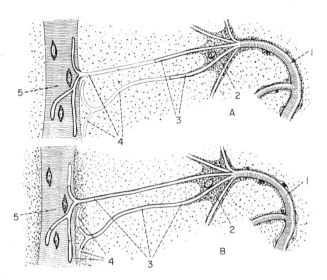

Fig. 7.9 Diagram of tracheal structure. 1. End of a tracheal branch; 2. Tracheoblast;
3. Air-filled portion of tracheoles; 4. Fluid-filled portion of tracheoles; 5. Muscle fibre.
A. In the resting state; B. During work—osmotic withdrawal of tracheolar fluid may
eventually allow air to penetrate right into the tissue. (Wigglesworth)[226]

in very primitive forms, linked on either side of the body by longitudinal tracheal
trunks. One or more pairs of spiracles often serve for inspiration and others more
anteriorly or more posteriorly, serve for expiration and there is effectively a
circulation of air through these longitudinal trunks (Fig. 7.10). In larger and more
active insects (e.g. bees and wasps) a deeper ventilation by air sacs further reduces the length of the passive gaseous diffusion pathway especially during
activity. This deep ventilation results from contraction of specialized abdominal
muscles, causing momentary occlusion of the air sacs. In this manner the tidal
volume may be raised to as much as 60% of the total air capacity, as in larvae of
Dytiscus. Control of spiracular opening and the presence of valves may also play a
part in increasing the effectiveness of this air circulation in the more superficial
parts of the system. During flight, when oxygen demand is high, ventilation is
enhanced by the action of the flight muscles in changing the shape and volume
of the thorax.

The main tracheae branch repeatedly and when the diameter is reduced to
about 2 to 5 μm, the branch commonly terminates in a stellate tracheal end-cell
or tracheoblast. Here abruptly arise a number of tracheoles which are less than
1 μm in diameter and are completely enclosed in a thin cytoplasmic sheath from
the tracheoblast. These terminate blindly, at variable lengths (200–350 μm) with
an ultimate diameter of about 0.2 μm, either on or between the cells of limb and
body wall muscles or other organs (Fig. 7.9). In the most active flight muscles the
tracheoles indent below the surface of the fibres and lie, enclosed in a sheath of

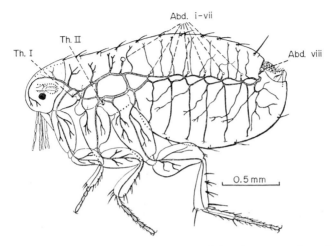

Fig. 7.10 Tracheal system of a flea, showing the left-hand representatives of two pairs of thoracic and eight pairs of abdominal spiracles together with a well-developed system of longitudinal tracheal trunks. (Wigglesworth)[226]

muscle plasma membrane, between the fibrils. It is no longer thought that tracheoles become intracellular within organs.[156]

Discontinuous release of carbon dioxide

As in other terrestrial animals regulation of ventilation is affected, in this case by control of spiracular opening, principally through variation in 'pulmonary' pCO_2 (see p. 147). In most insects exchanges of oxygen and carbon dioxide with the external air keep in step but in forms which are highly adapted to arid environments (e.g. *Tenebrio*, the mealworm; diapausing silkworm pupae; hibernating larval and adult Lepidoptera; beetles; cockroaches and locusts[156]) discontinuous release of carbon dioxide is found. This is thought to result from the phenomenon of spiracular fluttering. For part of the time the spiracles are kept so tightly closed that they are nearly gas-tight. Gas exchange in the tracheoles then takes place in a fixed volume of gas. Since oxygen uptake normally exceeds carbon dioxide output (to a greater or lesser degree according to the RQ) the pressure within the closed system falls. As the gaseous pO_2 falls, the spiracles are opened slightly in a fluttering manner and there is an inrush of air. In the face of this stream, carbon dioxide and water vapour are effectively prevented from diffusing outwards. Only periodically (at intervals which may be in extreme cases as long as 7 hours) do the spiracles open widely for a short time so that diffusion equilibrium can occur and the accumulated carbon dioxide escape in significant amounts. Direct experimental evidence in support of this hypothesis has been obtained in the diapausing pupa of the silk moth, *Hyalophora*.[142]

Regulation of tracheal respiration

Control of exchange with the tissues is regulated by two remarkable phenomena which were initially demonstrated and investigated by Wigglesworth.[226] In the short-term, increased demand for oxygen is facilitated by the accumulation of acidic metabolites in the tissues. The cellular fluid is thus rendered hypertonic to the extra-cellular fluid which fills the terminal parts of the tracheoles and a form of osmotic uptake of the tracheolar fluid occurs.* This has the effect of bringing the air/fluid interface within the tracheole closer to the respiring cells and thus shortening the final pathway of diffusion of oxygen in solution. As the acidic metabolites are eliminated when more aerobic conditions are established, the process is reversed. This regulatory mechanism is analogous to the opening-up of the capillary bed in other animals.

Long-term increases in demand for oxygen in particular parts of the body are met by an equally remarkable adaptive growth of the distribution and density of tracheae and tracheoles. Following section of tracheae or the implantation of organs, tracheoles are pulled by epithelial cell filaments into the oxygen deficient area. Such adjustment occurs before the next moult. Tracheae will also develop into hypoxic areas such as implanted organs, regenerating limbs etc., or will generally hypertrophy in animals kept at low pO_2. These tracheal developments only occur after the next moult.[226]

Size limitations

Although diffusion of oxygen in the gas phase is some 3×10^5 times faster than in aqueous solution, it still becomes severely limiting over long distances in narrow tubes. The insect tracheal system therefore has the inherent disadvantage of imposing a comparatively low limit to body size—a fact of which some science fiction writers seem to be unaware. The largest extant insects are tropical beetles which attain lengths up to 15 cm; they are able to grow to larger sizes than temperate forms because at the higher ambient temperatures at which they live, gaseous diffusion is correspondingly faster. Although tropical dragonflies with wing spans up to 2 feet occurred in Carboniferous times they had, like their modern relatives, very attenuated cylindrical bodies which were not more than 3 cm in diameter.

Krogh[126] made notable contributions to the diffusion theory of the tracheal system. The aggregate cross-section area usually remains almost the same at each level in the branching system, so diffusion is simply related to the distance from

---

* At least for the larva of *Aedes*, this is an over-simplification. The tracheolar fluid is thought to be dilute lymph and its level in the tracheole depends on the balance between capillarity and the imbibition force of colloids in the cytoplasm of the tracheoblast. The latter changes with tissue osmotic pressure.[226]

the spiracles. In the large larva of the goat moth *Cossus* the average tracheal length is 6 mm and the aggregate cross-section is 6.7 mm^2 and it was calculated that the animal's need for 0.3 mm^3 of oxygen per second could be supplied by diffusion without ventilation if there was a pO_2 difference of as little as 11 mm.

A ten-fold increase in linear dimensions would allow a ten-fold increase in diffusion rate for the same pO_2 difference but the animal's weight would be 1000 times greater and the metabolism at least 100 times greater ($\alpha W^{\frac{2}{3}}$). Oxygen can, of course, be supplied at much higher rates than 0.3 mm^3/sec in flying insects of modest size by exploiting the larger pO_2 difference which is always available and by reducing the passive diffusion pathway through active ventilation. Beyond this there is no evidence that any but passive diffusion processes are at work or are called for.

Aquatic adaptations

The insect tracheal system evolved essentially as an air-breathing mechanism but it has been adapted successfully for aquatic life a number of times. One kind of modification is represented by the tracheal gills on the abdomen of nymphal Plecoptera and Ephemeroptera and larval Trichoptera. Instead of opening to the external medium via a series of spiracles, closed and compression resistant tracheae ramify extensively within thin-walled expansions of the body wall. Irrigation is effected by rhythmic movements of the gills through the water. In some larval Odonata (e.g. *Aeschna*) an alternative site is found; the closed tracheae are found inside elaborate gill-structures, developed from the hind-gut lining, which are regularly irrigated. A third alternative for aquatic respiration via tracheal systems is discussed in the next section.

'Physical' gills

A considerable number of adult aquatic insects, mainly bugs and beetles, have adopted the habit of diving with an air bubble trapped by some part of the external body surface (e.g. below the elytra of beetles) in such a position that it communicates with one or more pairs of normal spiracles. The retention and renewal of the bubble is facilitated by appropriate distribution of hydrofuge hairs.

The bubble is frequently called an air-store and as such might be regarded as the insectan equivalent of the lung in pulmonate snails. However, it is clear that in many cases this conveys a quite misleading idea of its function and the term 'physical gill' (due to the Dutch comparative physiologist, H. J. Jordan) is to be preferred. Understanding of the role of the physical gill rests on a simple theoretical physical concept but it is not easy to demonstrate directly that such a principle is operating in practice. Nevertheless, indirect investigations have established such a role in a number of specific cases and it is probably operating similarly in many more.

If a volume of air is retained in contact with some gas-permeable surface of an animal on the one hand and with the aqueous external medium on the other, oxygen will be taken up from the bubble and carbon dioxide excreted into it. The carbon dioxide will rapidly disappear from the gas phase by solution in the water and the bubble will tend to shrink. In consequence, the varying conditions in the bubble may be described in terms of the volumes and partial pressures of oxygen and nitrogen alone. Uptake of gaseous oxygen has two effects: (a) a reduction in the volume of the bubble and (b) a change in the relative proportions of oxygen and nitrogen. Since the total pressure in the bubble remains the same, the changed proportions result in a decrease in pO_2 and an increase in pN_2. The bubble will therefore tend to a state of disequilibrium with the surrounding water which will be resisted by diffusion between the two phases, nitrogen tending to diffuse out and oxygen to diffuse into the bubble.

Now the extent to which equilibration will be at the expense of the movement of one gas as against the other will depend on the relative proportions of the two gases in the bubble and on the readiness with which each can cross the air/water interface (the so-called 'coefficient of invasion'). On both counts inward movement of oxygen is favoured relative to loss of nitrogen and in consequence, uptake of oxygen by the animal from the bubble is balanced by invasion of oxygen from the water. However, the bubble does slowly shrink due to loss of nitrogen. This air-breathing respiratory organ is thus assured of a supply of gaseous oxygen (even though the animal remains submerged) but only so long as there is gaseous nitrogen present in the bubble to act as a receptacle for the invading oxygen. Before the nitrogen finally disappears the area of bubble in contact with the water will fall to a level inadequate for the necessary rate of oxygen uptake. By then the animal will normally have made its way to the surface to replenish the bubble; functionally most important in this act is the collection of more nitrogen.

That the air bubbles carried by aquatic insects do function in this manner has been clearly established in a number of cases. It needs to be shown that (a) the animal (incapable of normal direct dissolved oxygen uptake) can be sustained for longer periods, in view of its known oxygen requirements, than can be accounted for by the initial oxygen content of the bubble; (b) that prolonged sustenance referred to in (a) does not occur if the animal's bubble is of pure oxygen.

The conditions governing the functioning and efficiency of the physical gill have been discussed and subjected to very careful experimental investigation by Wolvekamp and co-workers.[190, 232] In addition to confirming such a function in various adult aquatic insects including *Notonecta*, *Corixa*, *Nepa*, *Naucoris* and *Hydrous*, they show that there may be considerable variation between animals and between seasons in the relative efficiency of the function. One of the most important factors governing efficiency is the presence of effective irrigation movements (provided by the legs) to ensure that the air/water interface is not stagnant.

It should perhaps be stated that not all air bubbles carried by insects act as physical gills; some, such as those of *Dytiscus*, are inadequately exposed to the water and probably serve as simple oxygen stores. In either case an additional hydrostatic function may be significant.

In principle, exploitation of a physical gill is not limited to tracheate animals. A 'pulmonary' air bubble exposed to the water could be used in a similar manner by other air-breathing aquatic animals such as pulmonate snails. Although such a suggestion has been made in relation to *Lymnaea pereger* and *Physa fontinalis*,[94] some populations of which live remote from the shore line of large lakes, no demonstration of the function has been made. Artificial arrangements of this nature might enable man to remain under water without recourse to compressed gas supplies other than a little nitrogen.

Plastron respiration

If the air bubble constituting the physical gill could maintain a constant volume, the total pressure of the contained gases would tend to fall as oxygen was consumed but the partial pressure of nitrogen would remain the same and continue in equilibrium with the nitrogen tension in the water. There would therefore be no tendency for this gas to diffuse outward and the physical gill function would continue indefinitely without the need of replenishing with air (nitrogen) from the atmosphere.

Relatively large air bubbles such as are found under the elytra or wings or entangled in bristles on various parts of the body, are not capable of resisting shrinkage and must, therefore, be replenished periodically. This is not the case with very thin air films which adhere to large parts of the body surface of a number of other aquatic bugs and beetles. These films, which give a silvery iridescent appearance to the body, are capable of resisting high hydrostatic pressures and of persisting indefinitely. Such a system is known as a 'plastron' and its indefinite physical gill function is called 'plastron respiration'.

In the bug *Aphelocheirus* the plastron has been developed to a state close to theoretical perfection, as shown by the very extensive investigations of Thorpe and Crisp. The air film is trapped in the thickness of the plastron pile, a regularly arranged covering of minute cuticular hairs which rise to a height of only about 5 μm above the epicuticle and have their tips turned over at an angle of 90°. The hairs number about 2.5×10^6 per mm², are spaced about 0.5 μm apart and have a diameter of about 0.2 μm. This air film, whose volume is minute, will withstand a pressure of 4 to 5 atmospheres before wetting of the cuticle occurs. Because of its extreme thinness, lateral diffusion of oxygen within the film will be relatively slow but the effective openings of the abdominal and thoracic spiracles are spread out over a considerable area on the ventral surface by the development of curious, arborizing, rosette-like structures which form fine channels in the exocuticle.

The resistance of closed tracheal systems to compression (abdominal and hindgut gills of ephemerid and dragonfly larvae) is equally important, otherwise the air would disappear from them for the same reasons as in the non shrink-resistant physical gill. Thorpe[211] has given a comprehensive summary of this work and reviewed the possible significance of the mechanism in many representatives of other groups including the Coleoptera, Trichoptera, Lepidoptera and Hymenoptera.

8 The Nature and Distribution of Respiratory Pigments

The development of efficient circulatory systems and respiratory organs are of great importance in ensuring an adequate quantity and partial pressure of oxygen at the tissue level. Possibly more important, because of the immense potential for specific adaptation to particular environmental circumstances, is the development of respiratory pigments.

DEFINITION

If defined in the broadest possible terms as coloured substances which subserve a respiratory function, these pigments include the cytochromes, the flavoproteins and other molecules well known to the biochemist, which mediate the final stages of oxidation within the cell by the part which they play in hydrogen acceptor systems. However, these are omitted from the present discussion and attention is confined to those molecules which, occurring in sufficient concentration to lend visible colour to an animal's body fluids or tissues, mediate the transfer of oxygen at the extracellular or intercellular level. In the simplest possible terms these predominantly circulating pigments increase the oxygen capacity of the blood and so boost the oxygen transport potential of the circulatory system independently of the rate of circulation. However, a reasonable understanding of the observed diversity of roles of these substances must rest on a rather more sophisticated examination of their nature, properties and activities.

By virtue of their discernible colours, respiratory pigments have been recognized in a great number and variety of animals but there seems to be no *a priori* reason why some colourless substances with similar oxygen binding properties should not remain to be discovered. Conversely, several coloured body fluid pigments (such as the vanadium chromogen of some ascidians and the manganese-containing 'pinnaglobin' of the lamellibranch *Pinna*) have been investigated without disclosing any respiratory function.

The currently recognized pigments of proved respiratory function may be grouped into four classes: the haemoglobins, the haemocyanins, the chlorocruorins and the haemerythrins—to put them in a rough order of importance in the animal kingdom. In the earlier literature a fourth term 'erythrocruorin' is sometimes used to distinguish the porphyrin-based pigments of invertebrates but, since it is now known that these do not differ essentially from the haemoglobins of vertebrates, the distinctive term is no longer used. It is unfortunate that the prefix 'haem' (originally simply meaning 'blood' but now used also in the present context to denote a precise chemical entity) may suggest chemical affinities which do not in fact exist. There is a close chemical similarity between haemoglobins and chlorocruorins which is not shared by either haemocyanins or haemerythrins.

DISTRIBUTION

The distribution of these pigments has often been reviewed (see Manwell;[147,149] D. L. Fox;[55] H. M. Fox and Vevers;[61] Prosser[175]) so we shall here be content with a summary. This attempts to be representative while emphasizing the varied nature of the distribution. Some of the examples of the absence of a pigment are of considerable interest and significance.

Haemoglobins

Haemoglobins are of course characteristic of the vertebrates and are, with the notable exception of some antarctic fishes,[192] present in the blood of all normal adults. The larvae of the eel and of the sand-eel (*Amodytes*) are normally without, as are also occasional specimens of adult amphibia (e.g. *Xenopus*).[41] Among the vertebrates these vascular pigments are invariably found in erythrocytes. In addition, haemoglobins (referred to as myoglobins) are found in muscle cells, generally in mammals and birds, sporadically in teleosts and elasmobranchs.

Among invertebrates, respiratory pigments occur in a very sporadic fashion. In some taxonomic groups they are very common, while in others only exceptional genera or even species show them. Perhaps the most consistent phylum is the Annelida. Freely dispersed haemoglobin occurs in the plasma of many families with closed circulatory systems and in some cases erythrocytes are found in the coelomic fluid as well (*Travisia, Terebella*). But in the Syllidae, Aphroditidae and Chaetopteridae neither vascular system nor coelom contains a pigment. Where a functional circulatory system is lacking, coelomic erythrocytes may be present (Capitellidae, Glyceridae, *Polycirrus hematodes* and *P. aurantiacus* or may be absent (*Polycirrus tenuisetis* and *P. arenivorus*). Haemoglobin also occurs in corpuscles in some other groups which lack a closed circulatory system, including a number of holothurians (*Thyone, Cucumaria*), echiuroids (*Urechis, Thalassema*) and phoronids. Large amounts of freely dispersed haemoglobin also occur in the Pogonophora.[150]

In the remaining phyla the occurrence of haemoglobin is fairly or very infrequent. It is unknown in the malocostracan crustacea but not uncommon in the Entomostraca (*Artemia, Daphnia, Triops, Apus*). Among insects only one haemocoelic pigment is known from the larvae of a number of chironomid midges. In the Mollusca a few pelecypods (*Solen, Arca, Pentunculus*) have haemoglobin in corpuscles and one gastropod (*Planorbis*) has the pigment in solution. A few nemertines and nematodes have haemoglobin in body fluids, while among protozoa haemoglobin has been identified in certain strains of the ciliates *Paramecium* and *Tetrahymena*.

Myoglobins

Tissue located myoglobins are even more diversely distributed and by no means restricted to muscle (see Fox[60]). Among invertebrate tissues most consistently endowed are the radular muscles of gastropods but body-wall muscles sometimes have them as well (polychaetes *Arenicola, Potamilla* and *Travisia; Urechis* and *Ascaris*). Eggs and ovaries contain haemoglobins in *Daphnia, Chironomus,* the polychaete *Scoloplos* and the sipunculid *Thalassema.* Finally, in some nemertines, some gastropods, in *Aphrodite, Thalassema* and *Chironomus* larvae haemoglobins are found in central nerve cords.

Chlorocruorins

The distribution of the other classes of pigments is more easily delineated. Chlorocruorins, which are closely related to haemoglobins, are found only in solution in the plasma and seem to be confined to four polychaete families: Sabellidae, Serpulidae, Chlorhaemidae and Ampheretidae. Within the serpulid genus *Spirorbis* species are found with chlorocruorin, with haemoglobin or with neither; one species of *Serpula* has blood containing both! The habitats of all these tubicolous forms appear to be similar.[59]

Haemocyanins and haemerythrins

Haemocyanins, like chlorocruorins, have never been found in corpuscles nor in tissue cells. Free dispersal in the plasma is limited to the chitons, prosobranch and pulmonate gastropods and the cephalopods among the molluscs and to Malacostraca and a few arachnids (*Limulus, Euscorpius*) among the arthropods. Haemerythrins have an even more restricted distribution and are known at present in small groups in four unrelated phyla: *Magelona* (a polychaete); probably most sipunculids; *Priapulus* and *Halicryptus* (priapulids); *Lingula* and *Glottidia* (brachiopods). In all these cases the pigment circulates in corpuscles. There may be myohaemerythrin in the sipunculid *Dendrostomum.*

Systematics

Since the lists of respiratory pigment distribution are as yet incomplete, it is probably premature to attempt any generalization about the systematics of these molecules. Nevertheless, it does seem likely that they are all polyphyletic in origin. This is not surprising in the case of the haemoglobins, since the structure of the universal prosthetic group, haem, is closely similar to those of the cytochromes which are found in nearly all aerobic cells. It is probably not a difficult task for natural selection to call forth haem if an oxygen-binding pigment assumes a selective advantage in the living conditions of any particular form. More puzzling is the development of the completely unrelated alternatives, haemocyanin and haemerythrin, in groups where the cytochromes were at hand. At the same time some of the more localized gaps in the distribution, such as the absence of radular myoglobin from the Fissurellidae among the gastropods, are very likely to represent a phylogenetic loss.

STRUCTURE AND FUNCTIONAL PROPERTIES

All four classes of pigment share one important structural attribute. They are all conjugated proteins (long polypeptide chains bearing a non-amino acid prosthetic group) in which the prosthetic group contains a metal. [There are of course many other conjugated proteins which do not have oxygen-binding properties.] Within any of the four classes the structure of the prosthetic group, in which the basic oxygen-binding property resides, is constant. This justifies the grouping together of, for example, many haemoglobins of great functional diversity. The structural basis for diversity of properties and of functions within the class is found in detailed differences in the polypeptide chains. Some knowledge of the nature of these molecules is necessary for an understanding of the diversity of their roles.

Haemoglobin and chlorocruorin

The remarkable X-ray diffraction studies of Kendrew and Perutz and their co-workers have greatly advanced our knowledge of the configuration of the polypeptide chains of haemoglobin. At the same time development of methods of amino acid sequence analysis have made possible the complete delineation of the chain structure in a number of haemoglobins and revealed the differences (sometimes very slight) in the sequence which exist between some of the haemoglobin variants which occur in man. These two lines of investigation have thrown considerable light not only on the mechanism of oxygen-binding but also on the manner in which changes in the oxygen equilibrium characteristics, permitting adaptation to changing needs within an animal group, may be effected by the natural selection of variations in the polypeptide chain. More detailed discussion of these polypeptide chains will be delayed until later (p. 92).

Haem, the prosthetic group of haemoglobins, is a metalloporphyrin with an atom of iron at the centre (Fig. 8.1). Chlorocruorins contain a very similar group, the only difference being the substitution of a formyl group for a vinyl group on one of the four pyrrole rings. This may account for the dichroic nature of chlorocruorin solutions, red in concentrated, green in dilute solution; to what extent other properties are influenced by this change is unknown. A number of metals could occupy the centre of the porphyrin ring but only the presence of iron, together with coupling to an appropriate polypeptide, gives a soluble product capable of reversible oxygen-binding. In this context reversible binding means that which can be reversed by simply lowering the pO_2—reductants being unnecessary.

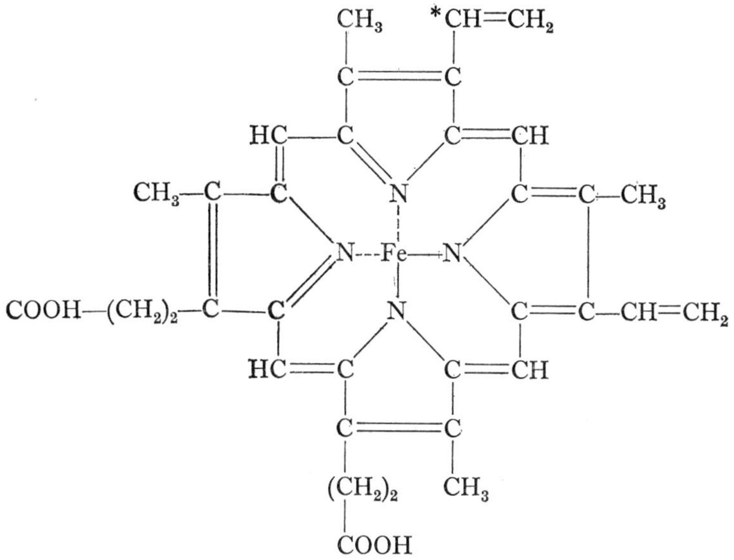

Fig. 8.1   The prosthetic group of haemoglobin. Four pyrrole rings are linked to form a porphyrin ring with an atom of ferrous iron at the centre. Two co-ordination bonds at right angles to the paper bind the iron to the polypeptide chain and to the molecule of oxygen or other ligand. The prosthetic group of chlorocruorin is identical except that a formyl group (C-CHO) is substituted for the vinyl group marked *.

In the functional pigment one molecule of oxygen is bound to the single ferrous ion via a co-ordinate bond on one side and to the polypeptide chain via the imidazole group of a histidine residue on the other side. A second co-ordinate bond links the Fe^{++} to the polypeptide chain, also by an imidazole group of a histidine residue (Fig. 8.6). Loss of the oxygen (possibly by replacement with water) involves only the redistribution of electrons, so the metal remains in the ferrous state and the process should be referred to as deoxygenation rather than reduction. Oxidizing agents can remove an electron from the iron but in this ferric state (methaemoglobin) the oxygen-binding property is lost. In this system the bound oxygen is called a ligand; other ligands which can be reversibly bound at the same site are nitric oxide and carbon monoxide.

Haemocyanin and haemerythrin

In the case of haemocyanin and of haemerythrin there is no evidence that the prosthetic group consists of more than the metal ions attached directly to the polypeptide chain; in neither case is the nature of the attachment residue known with certainty, though – SH groups are probably involved. The manner of oxygen-binding in these two pigments is also somewhat uncertain. One molecule is bound by two copper atoms on each polypeptide unit of haemocyanin; both are in the cuprous state before the attachment of oxygen but on oxygenation one may lose an electron to become cupric, so the process is possibly, in part, one of oxidation. Two iron atoms are associated with one molecule of oxygen in haemerythrin; in the deoxygenated state both are ferrous while on oxygenation both may become ferric.[118]

Oxygen-binding

In order to explain a number of observed changes in physico-chemical properties on oxygenation (including magnetic moments and absorption spectra) Manwell and others have postulated resonating systems for all the pigments. The following is taken from one of Manwell's excellent reviews[149] to which the reader is recommended for a much fuller treatment of the question of oxygen-binding and other physico-chemical topics.

$$\text{Fe(II)} \ldots \text{O}_2 \qquad \text{Fe(II)} \!\!-\!\! \text{O}_2$$

oxyhaemoglobin and oxychlorocruorin

$$\text{Cu(I)} \ldots \text{O}_2^- \!\!-\!\! \text{Cu(II)} \quad \text{Cu(I)} \ldots \text{O}_2 \ldots \text{Cu(I)} \quad \text{Cu(II)} \!\!-\!\! {}^-\text{O}_2 \ldots \text{Cu(I)}$$

oxyhaemocyanin

$$\text{Fe(III)} \!\!-\!\! {}^-\text{O}_2^- \!\!-\!\! \text{Fe(III)}$$
$$\text{Fe(II)} \ldots \text{O}_2^- \!\!-\!\! \text{Fe(III)} \qquad\qquad\qquad \text{Fe(III)} \!\!-\!\! {}^-\text{O}_2 \ldots \text{Fe(II)}$$
$$\text{Fe(II)} \ldots \text{O}_2 \ldots \text{Fe(II)}$$

oxyhaemerythrin

Manwell argues that these resonance schemes could resolve many apparently contradictory lines of evidence bearing on the question of oxygen-binding by haemocyanin and haemerythrin and remove the need to postulate true oxidation.

Three simple types of oxygen-binding as postulated by Klotz and Klotz, may be summarized by the scheme in Fig. 8.2 taken from another useful review by

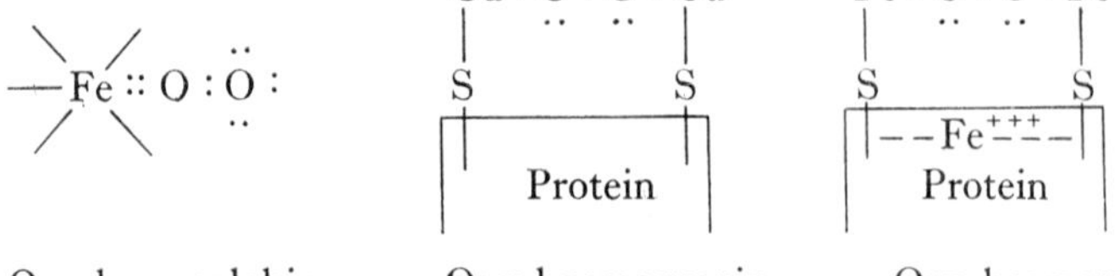

Oxy-haemoglobin   Oxy-haemocyanin   Oxy-haemerythrin

Fig. 8.2 Simplified summary of the types of oxygen-binding proposed for the blood pigments by Klotz and Klotz[118]. Chlorocruorin binds in the same manner as haemoglobin. The third ferric atom of haemerythrin which is not involved in oxygen binding is no longer thought to exist. (Manwell[149])

Wolvekamp.[233] Whatever the truth about oxidation may prove to be, and ideas about this are bound to change as X-ray studies of structure advance (p. 93), the use generally of the terms oxygenation and deoxygenation is to be preferred since they serve to remind us of the nature of the reversibility.

Oxygen equilibrium

Whatever its nature, oxygenation is a function of the pO_2 with which the pigment is in equilibrium, high pO_2 driving the equilibrium to the right and low pO_2 driving the equilibrium to the left:

$$Hb + O_2 \rightleftharpoons HbO_2$$

The proportion of the total haemoglobin (or other pigment) molecules in the oxygenated state (percentage saturation) is related to the pO_2 in a relatively complex manner, compared with the relation between pO_2 and dissolved oxygen concentration which is strictly linear. The relationship is normally represented after experimental determination by an oxygen equilibrium curve, usually by tradition and less correctly called an oxygen dissociation curve. Applying the Law of Mass Action to the simple equation above, we have:

$$\frac{[HbO_2]}{[Hb] \times [O_2]} = K \quad \text{or} \quad \frac{[HbO_2]}{[Hb]} = K \times [O_2]$$

With a given amount of pigment and a fixed value ascribed to K, the equilibrium constant, variation in the proportions of oxygenated to deoxygenated pigment yield values of $[O_2]$ or pO_2 such that the percentage saturation/pO_2 curve forms part of a rectangular hyperbola which is asymptotic to the 100% saturation level (curves 1 or 5 in Fig. 8.3). Alternatively in simple descriptive terms: in a system at low pO_2 with a fixed amount of pigment mostly in the deoxygenated state, the chance of an oxygen molecule striking an unoccupied binding site is relatively high. As percentage saturation increases, the chance of any one molecule colliding with one of the diminishing number of unoccupied sites is progressively reduced, so that increasingly large numbers of oxygen molecules are required to effect each increment in the saturation of the pigment; an asymptotic curve must result.

Carefully determined oxygen dissociation curves for any of the four classes of pigment fit fairly closely to an equation proposed by Hill:*

$$y = 100 \frac{kx^n}{1 + kx^n}$$

where y is % of pigment in oxygenated form (i.e. % saturation); x is the equilibrium pO_2; k is a constant representing the oxygen affinity of the pigment; and n is the 'sigmoid coefficient'.

* Based on certain assumptions which later proved incorrect, Hill's equation does not well fit the extreme ends of the observed curves; Manwell[147] therefore suggests that it be called Hill's approximation.

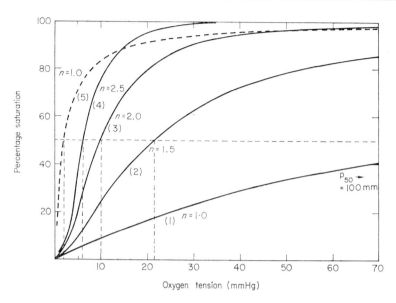

Oxygen tension (mmHg)

Fig. 8.3 Oxygen dissociation curves calculated from Hill's equation: $y = 100 \; kx^n /$ $(1 + kx^n)$ to illustrate the increasingly sigmoid nature as n increases. In contrast to the customary method of presenting such a family of curves, k has been kept constant at 0.01 except in the case of the dashed hyperbola where $k = 0.5$

The hyperbolic type of curve, obtained by applying the Mass Action Law to the simple equilibrium equation above or by making $n = 1$ in Hill's equation, is relatively uncommon in practice. The majority of observed curves are more or less sigmoid (curves 2, 3 and 4 in Fig. 8.3) and involve n values greater than 1. This reflects the fact that the simple equilibrium equation already given is an inadequate description of the system. For example, in virtually all vertebrate bloods the functional haemoglobin molecule is an aggregate of four units each of which consists of prosthetic group and polypeptide chain (Fig. 8.6) and the equilibrium equation accordingly should be written thus:

$$Hb_4 + 4O_2 \rightleftharpoons Hb_4O_2 + 3O_2 \rightleftharpoons Hb_4(O_2)_2 + 2O_2 \rightleftharpoons Hb_4(O_2)_3 + O_2 \rightleftharpoons Hb_4(O_2)_4$$

Each reaction in this sequence may have a different equilibrium constant because the binding of oxygen at any one site may influence the ease of binding at subsequent sites. There is fairly good evidence that in mammalian bloods the most significant change in the equilibrium constant follows the occupation of the first three sites (see Manwell[147] p. 208).*

* There has been very extensive study of the kinetics of the reactions of haemoglobin and other pigments with various ligands. Since the rates of association and dissociation of oxygen are very high and are not likely to be of significance in limiting normal physiological functions, this field will not be discussed. References may be found in the reviews of Antonini[5] and Roughton.[246]

Haem-haem interactions

These influences are known as haem-haem interactions and are almost always positive, i.e. later bindings are facilitated by earlier ones. In consequence, the dissociation curve is at all stages steeper than it would otherwise be and actually starts with a concave slope (Fig. 8.3). The degree of sigmoidness, represented by the value of n in Hill's equation, is a measure of the intensity of these interactions. The n value for observed dissociation curves can be obtained by taking values of x and y and substituting in the linear transformation of Hill's equation; when $\log (y/100y)$ is plotted against $\log x$ the slope of the resulting straight line equals n.

The common method of illustrating the influence of the n-number, by a family of curves lying more and more to the right as n increases, confuses the issue because it is not made clear that in such a series large progressive reductions in the value of k are also required. The family of curves in Fig. 8.3 were calculated from Hill's equation with (except for curve 5) a constant value of k; it will be seen that the sequence of curves is from right to left as n increases, i.e. increasing n also increases oxygen affinity (see below).

The degree of sigmoidness is not necessarily proportional to the number of units in the aggregated functional molecule. Thus the 4 unit haemoglobins of mammals show $n = 2.4$ to 2.9 while the 4 unit haemoglobin of the spiny dogfish, *Squalus suckleyi*, shows $n = 1$; the haemoglobins of *Arenicola marina* and *Eupolymnia* sp. each with around 200 units show $n = 4$ and 1 respectively.[147] As already seen, single unit haemoglobins lacking any possibility of haem-haem interactions must show $n = 1$. The other classes of pigment exhibit prosthetic group interactions of a similar nature.

The size of these aggregations is considered on p. 94 and their functional significance discussed on p. 95. The exact nature of the interactions is still a matter of debate and beyond the scope of the present survey. The reviews of Antonini[5] and of Riggs[186] may be consulted. However, it cannot be doubted that haem-haem interactions and other factors which influence oxygen affinity would be inoperative if the binding sites were widely separated from each other and from potentially 'influential' parts of the polypeptide chain; hence the importance of the close interlocking of the chains into a globular whole. The fact that n values do not exceed 6 even in the largest aggregations is probably due to the spatial limitation of these influences.

Oxygen affinity

The interaction between binding sites in only one of several factors which influence the *oxygen affinity* of a pigment. Even when n values remain the same the pigments of different animals reach particular saturation levels at different pO_2's (Fig. 8.4) so that when low levels of pO_2 are required (curve a) we speak of high oxygen affinity; when high levels of pO_2 are required (curve c) we speak of low oxygen affinity. This relative concept is conventionally quantified by quoting

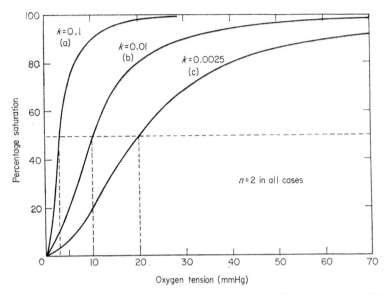

Fig. 8.4   Three oxygen dissociation curves calculated from Hill's equation: $y = 100kx^n / (1 + kx^n)$. In each case $n = 2$ but the values of k are varied, so that p_{50} values are 3, 10 and 20 mm respectively, i.e. oxygen affinity is *decreasing*

the pO_2 for 50% saturation (p_{50}); additional reference to p_{95} is useful, since p_{50} and p_{95} can vary independently from pigment to pigment unless n is the same. P_{95} and p_{50} are often referred to as 'loading tension' and 'unloading tension' respectively. These terms are preferably avoided since they may appear to imply that these are the tensions at which blood is actually loaded and unloaded *in vivo*, whereas they are no more than a useful conventional shorthand for describing the dissociation curve.

The basic aspect of oxygen affinity (i.e. apart from haem-haem interactions) is normally a species-specific property, determined by the influence of groups in the polypeptide chain upon the equilibrium constants of the reactions at individual binding sites and represented collectively by k in Hill's equation. High values of k indicate high oxygen affinity, n being equal (Fig. 8.4). It is self-evident that oxygen affinity must not be confused with *oxygen capacity* which, expressed as the volume of oxygen bound by the fully saturated pigment found in 100 ml of blood (vols%), is simply a measure of the effective pigment concentration.

Carbon monoxide affinity

The concept of affinity also applies to other ligands which may be bound by the prosthetic group (p. 83) and another variable between specific pigments is the relative affinity of the binding site for one ligand as against another. Most haemoglobins have a substantially higher affinity for carbon monoxide than for oxygen. A relatively low pCO will therefore effectively prevent oxygen-binding; hence the danger of carbon monoxide poisoning and the merit of administering pure oxygen in its treatment. Some values representing CO-affinity/O_2-affinity are given in Table 8.1. The ratios show a wide variation and are notably very low

Table 8.1   Relative affinities for carbon monoxide and oxygen of various respiratory pigments. The values are for $K = \dfrac{pO_2 \times (COHb)}{pCO \times (O_2Hb)}$. (From Prosser[175] except Ascaris[134])

Branchiomma (chlorocruorin)	570
Chironomus	400
Horse	280
Man	230
Arenicola	150
Tubifex	40
Planorbis	40
Rabbit	40
Various myoglobins	28–51
Ascaris body wall	0.82
perienteric fluid	0.08
Gasterophilus	0.67
Cytochrome oxidase	0.1

for the haemoglobins of Ascaris and Gasterophilus larvae; in these two genera oxygen affinity itself is exceptionally high (p. 142, 143).

Haemocyanin and haemerythrin were thought not to bind carbon monoxide because this gas is a reducing agent tending to donate rather than accept electrons and hence would not satisfy the properties for binding at the oxidation sites of these two pigments.[234] However, if the resonance schemes for ligand-binding (p. 84) operate, oxidation need not be invoked and carbon monoxide could in theory be bound. Furthermore, two investigators[187] have claimed that the haemocyanins of Limulus and Octopus respectively do have a low affinity for carbon monoxide. Manwell ([149] p. 69) advances reasons why the affinities of haemocyanins and haemerythrins for carbon monoxide should be low compared with their affinities for oxygen.

Temperature and oxygen affinity

While the basic oxygen affinity of any pigment, with or without the modifying effect of prosthetic group interactions, is genetically determined, there are additionally several normal environmental variables which often modify the relationship between percentage saturation and pO_2. Thus it is almost universally found that increase of temperature displaces the dissociation curve to the right. This is the simple consequence of the exothermic nature of oxygen-binding processes.

As Wolvekamp has pointed out ([232] p. 19), the increased oxygen requirements of poikilotherms at higher temperatures may be facilitated by the decrease in oxygen affinity and consequent easier unloading. The same may be true for homoiotherms also since body temperature may rise by 2 or 3 degrees in extreme activity. However, in either case excessive displacement of the upper end of the dissociation curve might endanger maximal loading in the respiratory organ ($p_{95} > p_{art}$). We have, moreover, already seen the difficulties which face aquatic poikilotherms in respect of ambient oxygen depletion and increased irrigation at higher ambient temperatures (p. 16). By way of compensation for these disadvantages, diffusion coefficients are slightly increased by rise of temperature (p. 4).

Carbon dioxide and oxygen affinity—The Bohr effect

Of much greater interest and functional significance is the influence of pCO_2 on oxygen affinity. This, the Bohr effect (after one of its discoverers), is now known to be a consequence of change in pH and so can also be induced normally by other acidic metabolites, such as lactic acid. When increase of pCO_2 or fall in pH moves the dissociation curve to the right, as is usually the case, the Bohr effect is said to be normal or negative (Fig. 9.2, p. 99). This is by far the commonest situation for pH changes within the physiological range. However, a few haemocyanins (including those of *Limulus polyphemus*, *Busycon canaliculatum* and *Helix pomatia*) exhibit reverse or positive Bohr effects in the presumed physiological range and a normal effect only in markedly alkaline regions.

The reversal of the Bohr effect has also been shown to occur in a number of 'normal' pigments (haemoglobin of *Rana catesbeiana*, *Squalus suckleyi*, *Eumetopias* (sea lion), rat and man; haemocyanin of *Homarus*) when studied in sufficiently acid conditions (Manwell[147] p. 210). In other words it is found that the p_{50}/pH relationship gives a curve with a pronounced maximum, as in Fig. 8.5. In most cases the physiological pH range falls across the descending part (– ve slope) of the curve, occasionally across the ascending part (+ ve slope).

There are also numbers of pigments in which the Bohr effect is apparently altogether lacking. These include haemoglobins of *Urechis caupo*, *Eupolymnia* (polychaete), *Polistotrema stouti* (hagfish), tadpole of *Rana catesbeiana*, haemerythrins of various sipunculids and the haemocyanins of some Amphineura. In these cases the p_{50}/pH relationship is a horizontal line (Fig. 8.5).

The magnitude of the Bohr effect is usually expressed as phi ($\phi = \Delta \log p_{50}/\Delta pH$). It is a genetically determined parameter which shows considerable adaptive variation. Some of these variations are discussed in the next chapter (p. 125). The extent of the change of p_{50} with change of pCO_2 depends not only on the genetic character of the pigment but also on the buffer capacity of the blood; in well-buffered bloods rather large changes of pCO_2 are required to change the pH sufficiently to alter p_{50} significantly.

The interpretation of these diverse Bohr effects at the molecular level presents great difficulties. The reader interested in this aspect should consult the reviews of Manwell[147,149], Riggs[186], Wolvekamp[233] and Antonini[5]. For present purposes

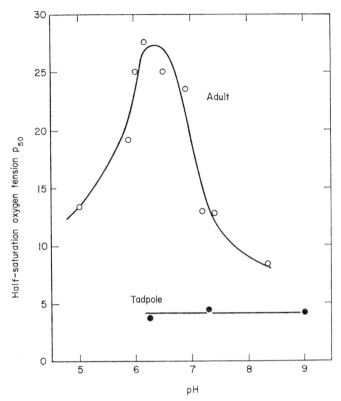

Fig. 8.5 Effect of pH on the oxygen affinity (measured as p_{50}) of the haemoglobin of the bullfrog adult and tadpole. The physiological pH range lies across the descending part of the curve (negative Bohr effect). (After Riggs[184])

it is sufficient to say that when a free H ion or proton from the dissociation of carbonic acid or other acidic metabolite is bound at some site on the polypeptide chain, the reduced negative charge on the protein molecule causes a change in the oxygen affinity of the oxygen-binding site. Manwell ([149] p. 91) has reviewed evidence suggesting that this interaction between oxygen-binding and proton-binding sites is fundamentally similar to the haem-haem interactions already discussed. As yet the nature of the proton-binding sites is not clearly established; in some cases there is good correlation between magnitude of the Bohr effect and the number of sulphydril groups; in other cases imidazole groups of histidine residues are implicated.

The Bohr effect represents one side of a reciprocal relationship. Just as bound protons normally hinder the binding of oxygen (negative Bohr effect), so bound oxygen normally hinders the binding of protons. Accordingly, deoxygenated blood will absorb more carbon dioxide for a given pCO_2 than oxygenated blood.

D

The functional significance of this, the Haldane effect, will be discussed in the section on carbon dioxide transport (p. 169).

The salt-effect

The form of the dissociation curve may also be markedly influenced by the salt environment in the blood. For example, the blood of *Helix pomatia* normally gives a very pronounced sigmoid curve while a salt-free (dialysed) solution of the haemocyanin gives a hyperbolic curve.[233] The oxygen affinity of a solution of human haemoglobin is some 10% higher in M/10 KCl than in M/10 NaCl.[175] Much work has been done on this 'salt-effect' and it is shedding some light on the mechanisms of pigment action. However, as yet there is little to suggest a biological significance in the observed behaviour so we shall not concern ourselves further with this aspect.

NATURE OF THE POLYPEPTIDE CHAINS AND THEIR AGGREGATIONS

We have seen some of the ways in which interspecific differences in the protein moiety affect the properties of respiratory pigments in each of the four classes. A fuller appreciation of the adaptive significance of these differences may arise if we now take a closer look at the nature of the polypeptide chains and their aggregations. As with other proteins, at least three levels of structure can be distinguished.

Primary structure

The primary structure is represented by the usual unbranched sequence of amino acids. Recent work involving controlled differential hydrolysis has led to a complete account of this sequence in several myoglobins and in a number of the haemoglobin variants found in man. It is known that in some of the abnormal haemoglobins very slight variations occur; e.g. HbS of (sickle-cell anemia) differs from the normal adult form (HbA) by the substitution of a single amino acid (a valine for glutamic acid) in the sequence of 146 constituting each of the β-chains (see below). Normal adult (HbA) and foetal (HbF) haemoglobins, on the other hand, differ from each other by about 40 substitutions on the β-chain, which are referred to as γ-chains.[38]

It is interesting to note that in the first 35 or so haemoglobin polypeptide sequences to be completely solved there are only seven absolutely invariable residues. Four of these are in contact with the haem group while two more (plus three for which only single exceptions are known) hold key positions in shaping the tertiary structure.[38]

Secondary, tertiary and quaternary structure

The coiling of the polypeptide chain in a typical α-helix gives the molecule a characteristic protein secondary structure for the greater part of its length. However, at particular points in the chain the helix is interrupted by irregular regions and sharp bends. These bends, most of which correspond to the positions of proline residues, give the molecule a compact shape and an irregular but specific tertiary structure, first revealed by the X-ray diffraction studies of Kendrew and his co-workers in 1957 on the myoglobin of the sperm whale. A representation of this molecule appears in Fig. 8.6; the haem group is seen attached to the thirty-seventh and ninety-third residues and lying in a shallow pocket.

Perutz and his collaborators[34] found that in haemoglobin the four chains consist of two identical pairs with slightly different structures at all three levels, the α- and β-chains. The β-chain is 7 residues shorter than the myoglobin chain but otherwise identical in configuration. The α-chain is a little shorter still and differs considerably in its detailed configuration. Nevertheless, the two pairs fit snugly together (two α above and two β below) to give a characteristic quaternary structure (Fig. 8.6).

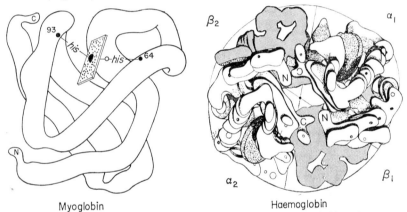

Myoglobin   Haemoglobin

Fig. 8.6 Representations of the tertiary structure of oxymyoglobin (left) and the tertiary and quaternary structure of haemoglobin (right). The sausage-like shape indicates the space occupied by the polypeptide chain. The haem group (rectangular) is attached to the chain by two of the iron atom (black ball) coordination bonds, one directly to the histidine residue 93 and one via the oxygen molecule to histidine residue 64; four other coordination bonds attach the iron atom to the porphyrin ring. There are many other interactions between the haem group side chains and the side chains of the amino acids lining the pocket in which the haem group lies; the latter are mainly non-polar groups giving the pocket a strongly hydrophobic character.

Vertebrate haemoglobins are tetramers of chains similar to that of myoglobin, represented here by layers of electron density 'contours' as determined by X-ray diffraction analysis (α-chains, white; β-chains, black). The view is from 'above', cf. 'side' view of myoglobin. The aggregation is held together by hydrophobic interactions between unlike chains ($\alpha_1\beta_2$, $\alpha_1\beta_1$, $\alpha_2\beta_2$, $\alpha_2\beta_1$). Haem groups, seen here as grey discs in α_1 and α_2 only, lie in pockets facing outwards on the hydrophilic surface of the aggregate. Oxygenation of one haem group results in a subtle but complex conformational change in the corresponding chain, which in turn influences the conformation of the corresponding residues in the other chains. These stereochemical changes could account for the Bohr effect and for haem-haem interactions.[244] (After Kendrew et al.[116] (myoglobin) and Perutz et al.[245] (haemoglobin).)

Two abnormal human haemoglobins have been found to lack the distinction between α- and β-chains. They are haemoglobin H with four β-chains and haemoglobin Bart's with four γ-chains. In each case the oxygen equilibrium resembles that of myoglobin, the oxygen affinity being low, the Bohr effect absent and the curve hyperbolic. It appears that vital functional characteristics of haemoglobin depend either upon the presence of α-chains or upon interactions between unlike chains.

Knowledge of the structure of haemoglobins is advancing at a very great rate and although the emerging models and concepts are highly complex they may be expected eventually to provide the key to all the basic properties which we have discussed and to the functionally important variations which will concern us later. For the present a very succinct account of the first steps in this direction and of some intriguing ideas about the evolution of haemoglobins may be found in the book by Dickerson and Geis.[38]

Polypeptide aggregations

In myoglobin, with a molecular weight of about 16 500, and in vertebrate haemoglobins (mol. wt. 65 000) the functional molecule consists of one* and four chains respectively, often known as monomers and tetramers. Invertebrate vascular haemoglobins, on the other hand, are aggregates of much larger numbers of units (each with a prosthetic group) of mol. wt. $15-20 \times 10^3$. Thus there are in *Daphnia* about 24 units, in *Planorbis* about 90, in polychaetes about 200. The only known exceptions are those of the lamellibranch *Arca*, which is in corpuscles, and of *Chironomus*, which is free in the haemocoel; these are 4 and 2 unit aggregates respectively. There is evidence that these larger aggregates are also characterized by a multiplicity of polypeptide types ([149] p. 60).

The other classes seem generally to occur as large aggregates. Haemocyanins fall into two groups, both with rather longer polypeptide chains. In arthropods the unit molecular weight is $c.\ 74 \times 10^3$ and the aggregates range from $c.\ 400 \times 10^3$ (*Pandalus*) to $c.\ 800 \times 10^3$ (*Homarus*). By contrast molluscan haemocyanins are built of smaller units ($c.\ 50 \times 10^3$) into larger aggregates ranging from $c.\ 2900 \times 10^3$ (*Octopus*) to 8900×10^3 (*Helix*). Data for the remaining classes are sparse but haemerythrin of the sipunculid *Golfingia* totals $c.\ 120 \times 10^3$ in units of 15×10^3, while that of *Sipunculus* apparently totals only 66×10^3. The chlorocruorin of *Sabella*, which has an aggregate mol. wt. of $c.\ 3400 \times 10^3$ (similar to polychaete haemoglobins), is said to be built from units of 35×10^3. Some evidence on the nature of the packing of these large aggregates is beginning to emerge from electron microscope studies which again indicate a basic difference between haemoglobins and haemocyanins; the packing of the former follows an hexamerous symmetry, of the latter, a pentamerous symmetry (Manwell[149] p. 60). These data are summarized in Table 8.2.

* Two unit myoglobins of mol. wt. $31-34 \times 10^3$ have been found in a number of gastropods.[209]

Table 8.2   A selection of approximate molecular weights of respiratory pigments with an indication of the probable unit polypeptide weight and number of units in the aggregate. (From data collected by Manwell[147, 148, 149] and Prosser[175])

	Pigment	Total and unit m.wt.		Location
Vertebrates generally	MyoHb	17 000	1	Muscles
Cyclostome *Lampetra*	Hb	17/34 000*	1(2)	Corpuscles
Polychaete *Notomastus*	Hb	36 000	2 × 18 000	Corpuscles
Midge larva *Chironomus*	Hb	34 000	2 × 17 000	Plasma
Vertebrates generally	Hb	68 000	4 × 17 000	Corpuscles
Lamellibranch *Arca*	Hb	72 000	4 × 18 000	Corpuscles
Sipunculid *Sipunculus*	Herythn	66 000	4 × 16 500	Corpuscles
Sipunculid *Golfingia*	Herythn	120 000	8 × 15 000	Corpuscles
Prawn *Pandalus*	Hcy	400 000	5 × 75 000	Plasma
Lobster *Homarus*	Hcy	800 000	10 × 75 000	Plasma
Branchiopod *Daphnia*	Hb	420 000	24 × 17 500	Plasma
Cephalopod *Octopus*	Hcy	2 800 000	56 × 50 000	Plasma
Gastropod *Helix*	Hcy	8 900 000	180 × 50 000	Plasma
Gastropod *Planorbis*	Hb	1 540 000	90 × 17 000	Plasma
Polychaete *Sabella*	Chlcr	3 400 000	98 × 35 000	Plasma
Polychaete *Arenicola*	Hb	3 000 000	180 × 17 000	Plasma

* In pure solution cyclostome haemoglobins are single units but inside the erythrocyte they behave as though there is a loose pairing of the molecules ([148] p. 409).

Functional significance of aggregation and of erythrocytes

It has long been recognized that intracellular pigments, whether in tissues or in circulating corpuscles, have low molecular weights, whereas extracellular pigments in free solution in body fluids have very high molecular weights. On the data at present available the dividing line comes at about 200×10^3. Freely dissolved pigments must be large molecules if they are not to be lost via excretory filters (mammalian haemoglobin in free solution may pass the glomerular filter). The haemoglobin of *Chironomus* with its mol. wt. of 34×10^3 is exceptional but so is the absence of any renal filtration. For coelomic pigments, enclosure within corpuscles seems to be necessary to prevent loss through coelomoducts or nephridia; in this case the molecular weight is low. The polychaete *Nephtys* provides an exception to prove this rule; here the coelomic pigment is freely dispersed but this genus lacks coelomoducts and has (closed) protonephridia.[105]

The inclusion of haemoglobin within corpuscles throughout the vertebrates is related to a complex of factors. If the pigment, of mol. wt. 66×10^3 and in sufficient amount to give an oxygen capacity of 20 vols %, were to circulate freely dispersed in mammalian blood, the colloid osmotic pressure would be about 175 mm, a figure quite incompatible with a reasonable water balance between tissues and blood. Alternatively, if the mol. wt. were large enough (c. 400×10^3) to reduce the colloid O.P. to an appropriate level without reduction of oxygen capacity, the viscosity of the blood would become impossibly high. In fact the oxygen capacity is achieved by packing the pigment at very high concentration into corpuscles, while the necessary colloid O.P. of about 30 mm is due to distinctive plasma proteins.

The more modest oxygen requirements of invertebrates can usually be met by much lower pigment concentrations and increase of mol. wt., (in order to keep colloid O.P. at a reasonable level and to prevent loss via excretory filters) can occur without excessively raising the blood viscosity. In the case of *Chironomus*, with an oxygen capacity up to 6 vols % and a mol. wt. of 34×10^3, the colloid O.P. must be of the order of 100 mm.

Corpuscular pigments are always of low molecular weight, even among representatives of groups in which large freely dispersed molecules are the rule (e.g. the polychaete *Notomastus*—36×10^3). So it is possible that where feasible within the confines of a corpuscle, a low molecular weight is in itself an advantage in some, as yet, unestablished way.

The blood corpuscle may also be regarded as a means of ensuring for the respiratory pigment an advantageous special environment. We shall later note (p. 134) some examples of the differences in properties of pigments of particular species studied in solution and in the intact corpuscle. These changes on release from the cell may involve oxygen affinity, Bohr effect and haem-haem interactions. In some cases the changes are elicited simply by haemolysis; in others the changes are only apparent after extensive dialysis (see Prosser[175] p. 213). The most obvious conclusion is that the ionic environment is of great importance in determining the precise oxygen-binding properties.

A fuller discussion of this topic is unnecessary at present but we should be warned that *in vitro* studies of respiratory pigments, designed to throw light on their normal physiological functions, should be made on fresh whole blood wherever possible, even when corpuscles are not involved. Finally, it has been suggested that the corpuscle increases the survival time of individual haemoglobin molecules in the face of certain oxidative processes which are liable to occur in the plasma.[135]

9 Transport Functions of Respiratory Pigments

Having reviewed the structure and general properties of respiratory pigments we may turn to an examination of the various ways in which they can expedite the supply of oxygen to the active tissues. Consideration of the general situation of a circulating pigment in relation to the diffusion picture presented in Chapter 2, will facilitate discussion of specific cases.

GENERAL TRANSPORT CONCEPTS

Loading and unloading—hyperbolic v. sigmoid curve

Fig. 9.1 shows two possible oxygen dissociation curves for a blood with an oxygen capacity slightly in excess of 4 vols% which is virtually fully saturated at 120 mm pO_2. For comparison, the linear relationship of oxygen solubility in the saline medium of the plasma is also shown. The pO_2 of the external medium is represented by point E on the abscissa, the condition of arterial blood by A at a pO_2 some 10 mm lower—the extent of the gradient across the respiratory epithelium. Suppose that in a moderate state of activity the needs of the tissue can be met if each 100 ml of blood passing through it gives up 1 ml of oxygen (1 vol% turnover). Then in the case represented by the sigmoid curve, venous pO_2 would have to fall to 50 mm, whereas for the hyperbolic curve it would be 30 mm. Both these venous pO_2s might well be adequate to deliver this amount of oxygen at the required rate down the final diffusion gradient from the capillary lumen to the more remote cells. If, however, the need for oxygen rises to 2.5 vols % then the final diffusion would begin at 25 mm pO_2 for the sigmoid curve, for the hyperbolic curve at only 8 mm which might well prove inadequate. Looking at the difference in another way, if the venous pO_2 were to remain at 50 mm the contributions of the two pigments would be 1.0 and 0.5 vols % respectively, while if the venous pO_2 were fixed at 25 mm the contributions would be 2.5 and 1.2 vols% respectively. In these two situations the dissolved oxygen alone would contribute only about 0.2 and 0.3 vols% respectively. Either pigment is superior to a system of dissolved oxygen transport alone, while that with the sigmoid curve is potentially able to deliver any part of its bound oxygen load at a higher pressure than that with the hyperbolic curve. The pigment with the hyperbolic curve can bind as much oxygen as that with the sigmoid curve but can only give up the major part of its load if venous pO_2 falls so low that the final diffusion delivery is inadequate.

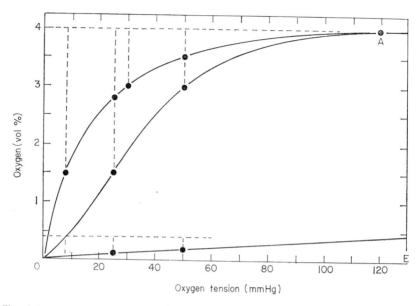

Fig. 9.1 Hypothetical comparison of the oxygen turnover possibilities of oxygen in solution against pigment transport with hyperbolic or sigmoid dissociation curves. Ambient pO_2 is assumed to be 130 mm (E) ; arterial pO_2 120 mm (A). The other points (●) to the left represent the various venous possibilities mentioned in the text; for each of these the oxygen turnover is shown by the vertical distance below the 4 vols % line (0.4 vols % in the case of dissolved oxygen). This figure also serves to illustrate the relationship between mammalian haemoglobin and myoglobin discussed on p. 135.

pO_2 buffering

By comparison with the dissolved oxygen system both the above-mentioned pigments effectively reduce the pO_2 drop needed to 'turn over' or liberate a given proportion of the total oxygen. By analogy with the familiar systems which buffer H ion concentration, we may therefore speak of respiratory pigments as pO_2 *buffers*. The effectiveness of this buffer system is indicated by the steepness of the curve and in Fig. 9.1 the terminal part of the hyperbolic curve is much the steepest. However, in functional terms the pO_2 range of the buffer is more important and here the sigmoid curve is likely to give the greatest advantage in the circumstances mentioned.

Allied to the basic improvement of oxygen-carrying capacity, this pO_2 buffer role is fundamental to the understanding of virtually all oxygen transport functions of respiratory pigments. There is also a sense in which the superior oxygen capacity of the blood itself constitutes a buffer system. Blood returns to the lung or gill at relatively low pO_2. If a pigment is lacking, only a rather small amount of oxygen diffuses across the epithelium before the blood comes to equilibrium with the external medium and the diffusion gradient disappears. But given a respiratory pigment (with or without haem-haem interactions) equilibration occurs only after a relatively large amount of oxygen has passed down the diffusion gradient.

Functional significance of the Bohr effect

It is clear that the presence of haem-haem interactions (sigmoid curve) is advantageous in allowing a high oxygen turnover at a relatively high venous pO_2 and the functional importance of the normal Bohr effect is to enhance this advantage. In Fig. 9.2 two dissociation curves are shown; they represent the oxygenation/pO_2 relationships for a single pigment at two different levels of pCO_2—those of arterial and venous blood respectively. Conditions as the blood leaves

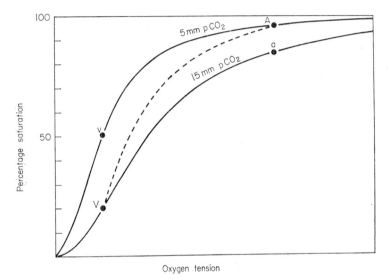

Oxygen tension

Fig. 9.2 Illustration of the functional significance of a hypothetical normal (negative) Bohr effect. Both curves were calculated from Hill's equation and are equally sigmoid ($n = 2$ in both cases) but represent different oxygen affinities (k being .01 and .0025 respectively). In practice change in pCO_2 (or pH) is often found to result in a change of n also. The effective dissociation curve is A-V.

the respiratory organ are defined by point A and as it leaves the tissue capillary bed, by point V. It is apparent that the effective dissociation curve is represented by the dotted line A-V and that the Bohr effect in this case increases the oxygen turnover by the amount V-v. While the uptake of carbon dioxide by the capillary blood moves the limit of oxygen dissociation to the lower curve, the loss of the carbon dioxide across the respiratory epithelium ensures that the limit of association lies once more on the upper curve. Such an arrangement is advantageous only so long as there is no tendency for pCO_2 to rise in the external medium;

D 2

if this were to happen in the above example the arterial condition might be represented by point a, the arterial blood failing to become fully saturated. Variations in the nature and extent of the Bohr effect are discussed later.

Potential scope for adaptation

As seen in Chapter 8, variations in the polypeptide structure of the pigment molecules result in changes in many physico-chemical properties. Functionally, the most important are basic oxygen affinity (defined by p_{50}), sigmoidness (n) and the extent of Bohr and temperature effects. Variations in these four parameters will account for almost all the observed differences between the respiratory pigments of different animals. Since the variations are genetically determined through the common mechanism of protein replication, the whole system provides a remarkably effective means of adaptation through normal processes of mutation and natural selection. Examination of a number of examples will serve to illustrate some very interesting adaptations to particular environments and the different kinds of role which respiratory pigments have come to fill in the animal kingdom.

HIGH TENSION OXYGEN TRANSPORT

The most familiar mode of oxygen transport, as found in mammals for example, involves movement from external media in which the pO_2 is consistently high, across an epithelium which presents only a modest barrier to diffusion. Arterial pO_2s are therefore not far removed from a high ambient level and venous pO_2s are also relatively high. Mediating such transport, pigments have an appropriately low oxygen affinity. This form is characteristic of all air-breathing vertebrates, which are assured of a consistently high level of alveolar pO_2, although the shortcomings of a tidal ventilation system do not usually allow this to rise above 100 mm. Birds achieve somewhat higher alveolar pO_2s as a result of their unusual ventilation arrangements (p. 67) and these are correlated with haemoglobins of unusually low oxygen affinity. A limited number of aquatic invertebrates whose habitat and mode of life similarly assure a consistently high level of external dissolved oxygen, also utilize low affinity pigments; high values of p_{50} are found in the polychaetes *Sabella*, *Nephtys*, and *Eupolymnia* and in the squid *Loligo*.

Because the ambient pO_2 and the diffusion barrier of the respiratory epithelium are consistent in such forms, arterial pO_2 will also be rather constant. It is therefore advantageous for the oxygen affinity to be adjusted so that the region of c. 95% saturation coincides with this arterial pO_2. If this so-called 'loading tension' considerably exceeded arterial pO_2 the pigment would never be fully saturated, while if it were significantly below the arterial level, part of the available diffusion gradient across the respiratory epithelium would be wasted. This adjustment, found in a number of animals which enjoy a consistently high ambient pO_2, is illustrated in Table 9.1.

Table 9.1   Relationship between arterial oxygen tension and the degree of saturation of arterial blood. In spite of very variable differences between ambient and arterial pO_2s, animals adapted to live at consistently high ambient pO_2 achieve high arterial percentage saturations because the oxygen affinities of their respiratory pigments are adjusted to individual needs. Notable exceptions to this generalization are the decapod crustacea represented by *Panulirus interruptus*. (Data from various authors as indicated)

	Arterial pO_2	Arterial % saturation
Sipunculid *Sipunculus nudus*[52]	32†	90
Echiuroid *Urechis caupo*[177]	75†	97
Gastropod *Busycon canaliculatum*[85]	36	95
Squid *Loligo pealei*[176, 178]	120	94*
Octopus *O. vulgaris*[227]	85*	97*
Lobster *Panulirus interruptus*[180]	7	54
Skate *Raja ocellata*[39]	70	93
Carp *Cyprinus carpio*[218]	85	93
Turtle *Chelydra serpentina*[85]	57	95
Duck[219]	102	98
Pigeon[219]	105	96
Goose[220]	94	96
Rabbit[12]	91	95
Horse[85]	100	98
Man[2]	100	97

* Not given by the original authors but calculated from their data.
† Coelomic pigments, where the arterial-venous distinction is absent.

Chlorocruorin in the sabellids

Amongst the best known of low affinity invertebrate pigments is the haemocyanin of *Loligo*—this is discussed later in relation to the Bohr effect (p. 126). Also fairly well understood, from the work of Fox,[56] is the case of the chlorocruorin of *Sabella*, the principal genus in a family of tubicolous polychaetes whose pigment distributional quirks were noted earlier (p. 81). In *S.* (*Spirographis*) *spallanzani* oxygen is bound to the extent of 10.2 vols % in equilibrium with 760 mm of oxygen but only 9.1 vols % with air. A similar failure to reach full saturation at atmospheric pO_2 is found in *S. pavonina* and *Branchiomma*. Unless these animals are frequently exposed to sea-water which is super-saturated with oxygen (and there is no evidence to suggest this), they would appear to represent a notable exception to our generalization about the adjustment of 'loading tensions'.*

Observed values of p_{50} for *S. spallanzani* range from 8 mm at pH 8 and 10°C to 29 mm at pH 7.4 and 26°C—the upper end of this pH range probably repre-

* No high affinity chlorocruorins have so far been discovered; it is therefore conceivable that very low oxygen affinity is a fixed characteristic of this group of pigments, in contrast to the variability of this property in the haemoglobins and haemocyanins.

sents conditions of actual unloading so venous pO_2s are likely to be relatively high. Unfortunately we know nothing of actual arterial and venous tensions; neither is it possible to make reasonable estimates of percentage saturation of the blood *in vivo*. However, Ewer and Fox[48] attempted to deduce something of the function of chlorocruorin in the related *S. pavonina* using the carbon monoxide method.

A simple comparison of the oxygen uptake *v.* ambient pO_2 relationship in normal animals and in those previously exposed to carbon monoxide to inactivate the haemoglobin (or chlorocruorin), should indicate the extent of the pigment's gas transport contribution. However, even with appropriate precautions (e.g. excessive pCO can inactivate cellular oxidases) there are some reservations about the method, which have been discussed elsewhere ([107] p. 74), and the results must be accepted with caution.

The oxygen consumption of CO-treated *Sabella* was approximately 33% less than that of normal animals over a range of external pO_2s from 150 mm down to 30 mm (Fig. 9.3d). Thus, in contrast to the pigments of very many invertebrates, the chlorocruorin of *Sabella* does appear able to mediate oxygen transport at high ambient tensions and this is entirely consistent with its low oxygen affinity.

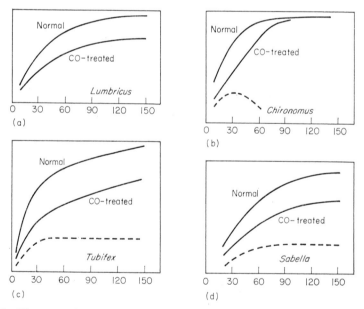

Fig. 9.3 Diagrammatic representation of the results of four studies using the CO-method. Abscissa scales represent dissolved oxygen tensions in mm Hg; ordinates represent oxygen consumption but not to the same scale. The dotted lines in (b), (c) and (d) represent the differences between normal and CO-treated animals. Note the distinction between the pattern for *Chironomus* and for the others. (Data from: (a) Johnson;[104] (b) Ewer;[47] (c) Dausend;[37] (d) Ewer & Fox[48])

Is this deduction consistent with the actual prevailing ambient conditions? Many tubicolous animals, by virtue of their mode of life, encounter highly significant periods of very low ambient pO_2 (see, for example, the discussion of *Chironomus*—p. 111) but in the sabellids the situation appears to be different. Oxygen uptake by the ciliated branchial crown is supplemented by transfer across the general body wall which, although enclosed by a tube of mud and mucus, is very effectively irrigated by peristaltic action of the body wall muscles. In his behaviour studies of the genus *Sabella*, Wells[224] found that generally, irrigation of the tube proceeds continuously even when the branchial crown is withdrawn. Irrigation pauses of up to 1 hr do occur in *S. pavonina* but provided that these do not coincide with withdrawal into the tube, there seems to be no reason why an adequate area of respiratory epithelium should not be continuously irrigated. Thus in this predominantly sub-littoral group, there should be no interruption of the supply of well-aerated water and a pigment suited to transport at high tensions in the blood is entirely appropriate.

Although not yet fully investigated, high tension transport seems to be the function of haemoglobin in another sedentary polychaete, the terebellid *Eupolymnia*.[146] In this pigment the hyperbolic dissociation curve shows a p_{50} of 36 mm at 10°C and the pigment is not fully saturated at atmospheric pO_2.

The case of the errant, burrowing polychaete *Nephtys* which is discussed later (p. 138), may also be included in the very limited list of invertebrates with low oxygen affinity pigments apparently adapted for high tension transport. However, the exploitation of consistently high ambient pO_2 is not always mediated by low affinity pigments as will be seen in the next section.

LOW TENSION TRANSPORT FROM HIGH AMBIENT pO_2

A number of investigations have shown that certain animals which enjoy a consistently high ambient pO_2 are provided with circulating pigments of high oxygen affinity. This situation arises because, unlike those mentioned above, these forms are characterized by exceptionally large diffusion barriers at the respiratory surface so that arterial pO_2s are low in spite of oxygen abundance in the immediate environment.

Decapod crustacea

As a group the decapod crustacea seem to belong to this category. Until recently it was even doubted whether the haemocyanins of crabs subserved an oxygen transport function at all, since some observations had shown that the total oxygen content of the blood was inferior to that of the surrounding sea-water. Redmond[180] first resolved this paradox with some observations which caused surprise at the time but clearly demonstrated for three species the importance of the pigment for life in well-aerated water. The essential features of this work are summarized in Fig. 9.4 and are included, for comparison with later studies, in Table 9.2.

Taking for example the spiny lobster *Panulirus interruptus* (not to be confused with the European *Palinurus*), we see that p_{50} and p_{95} are 6.3 and 25 mm,

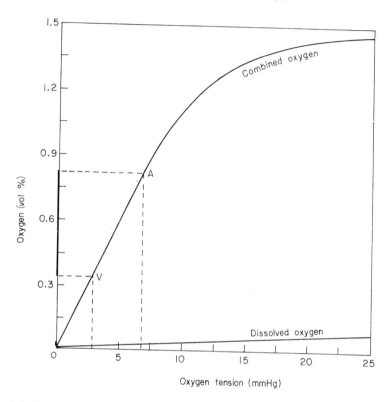

Fig. 9.4   Respiratory cycle in the spiny lobster *Panulirus interruptus*. The importance of the haemocyanin is indicated by the comparison of the turnover of combined and dissolved oxygen (thickened portions of the ordinal scale) which occurs in animals living in air-saturated sea-water Points A and V represent the state of arterial (pericardial, pO_2 7 mm) and venous (abdominal sinus, pO_2 3 mm) blood respectively. (Redmond[180])

representing a much higher oxygen affinity than in the cases discussed above and seemingly ill-suited to an animal living in air-saturated water. However, determination of arterial (pericardial) and venous (abdominal sinus) pO_2s gave values of only 7 and 3 mm respectively. In these conditions arterial haemocyanin was 54% saturated, 96% of the total oxygen content of 0.82 vols % being bound; in venous blood 22% saturation was found, 97% of the total 0.35 vols % being bound. The total A-V oxygen turnover of 0.47 vols % is almost exactly the amount which the blood could dissolve if equilibrated with air-saturated water but, because of the conspicuous failure of arterial blood to come to equilibrium with the external medium, about 96% of the turnover is mediated by the pigment. Thus,

Table 9.2 Oxygen capacities and arterial and venous blood parameters in the bloods of some decapod crustacea. In each case the *in vivo* gas measurements were made on freshly drawn blood from animals in well-aerated water. (Data from Redmond[180, 181, 183] except for last two species from Spoek[203])

Species	A-V	p_{50} mm	Oxygen capacity vols% Bound	Oxygen capacity vols% Soln.	T °C	*In vivo* O_2 content Total O_2 vols%	*In vivo* O_2 content Hcy %satn.	*In vivo* O_2 content pO_2 mm	*In vivo* O_2 content %O_2 as O_2Hcy	*In vivo* CO_2 pCO_2 mm	*In vivo* CO_2 A-V pH
Panulirus interruptus	A	6	1.53	0.46	15	0.82	54	7.0	96	5.0	.02
	V					0.35	22	3.0	97	5.3	
Loxorhynchus grandis	A	5	0·58	0.45	14	0.41	68	8.0	90	18.0	.01
	V					0.17	30	3.0	94	18.5	
Homarus americanus	A	5	0.86	0.45	14	0.44	49	5.3	95	2.3	.03
	V					0.18	20	2.3	95	2.5	
Cardisoma guanhumi	A	4	2.43	0.40	29	1.66	68	5.7	99		
	V					0.90	33	3.2	99		
Gecarcinus lateralis	A	18	1.72	0.45	26	1.45	81	29.0	94		.06
	V					0.61	36	14.0	94		
Maia squinado	A	19	0.74		21	0.54	61	24.4	84	1.3	
	V					0.33	33	18.3	81	3.1	
Homarus gammarus	A	10	0.94		20	0.61	67	14.9	91	3.3	
	V					0.31	29	8.2	89	3.7	

despite the rather low oxygen capacity (c. 1.5 vols%) of the pigment and its failure to reach more than 54% saturation in the gills, transport of oxygen is some 25 times more effective with the pigment than without it. Similar conclusions are suggested by somewhat less extensive data obtained by Redmond for the sheep crab *Loxorhynchus grandis* and the lobster *Homarus americanus*.

Later, Redmond[181] found that in the land crab *Cardisoma guanhumi* the oxygen affinity of the haemocyanin is even higher and the arterial pO_2 lower, so that the marked saturation deficiency persists. Spoek[203] made similar observations of the crab *Maia squinado* and the lobster *Homarus gammarus* (formerly *H. vulgaris*) which entirely supported Redmond's findings. He found appreciably lower oxygen affinities in these species together with higher arterial and venous pO_2s but the general picture was essentially the same and as before, the saturation of the arterial blood pigment was strikingly deficient. Finally, Redmond[183] found a further pigment of somewhat lower oxygen affinity in another land crab, *Gecarcinus lateralis*, where arterial blood was 81% saturated at a pO_2 of 29 mm. Even here the gradient across the respiratory epithelium considerably exceeds 100 mm. In all these examples (Table 9.2) we find a consistent picture of relatively high affinity pigments apparently adapted for transport from high ambient pO_2 but at low internal tensions, an arrangement which is necessitated by very inefficient transfer across the respiratory epithelium.

One set of discordant results should be mentioned. Zuckerkandl[240] found variation of haemocyanin and oxygen content of arterial blood during the moulting cycle in *Maia*. In attempting to calculate arterial pO_2 indirectly, he used a suspect early dissociation curve. Had he used Spoek's dissociation curve, Zuckerkandl's arterial pO_2s would have been consistent with the rest. Spoek's figures and Redmond's for *Gecarcinus* are the only blood pO_2s determined directly in crustacea.

If this general picture is a true one, it may well be asked why these crustacea consistently fail to make full use of the oxygen-binding capacity of the available pigment. Redmond himself[180] suggested the reserve capacity might be used at lower temperatures (when a normal temperature effect would move the curves to the left) if arterial pO_2s remained the same. Certainly all the data cited were obtained at temperatures well above the minima of the respective seasonal ranges.

On the other hand, if the data are summarized, as a series of dissociation curves (Fig. 9.5), an alternative highly speculative explanation suggests itself. In all cases the arterial-venous cycle is confined to the steepest part of the curve and a functionally sufficient oxygen turnover is achieved with minimal change of pO_2. Thus the pO_2-buffering action of the pigment is being exploited to the maximum extent, not only keeping the venous pO_2 up but also keeping the arterial pO_2 down. With normally adapted dissociation curves (p_{95} roughly corresponding to arterial pO_2—see Table 9.1), once these pigments had reached full-saturation, a comparatively small additional diffusion of oxygen into the blood (adding only to the dissolved oxygen load) would tend to raise arterial pO_2 to much higher levels than are actually found, especially at lower temperatures. If the system is adapted to keeping down arterial pO_2 at all costs, we may seek the explanation

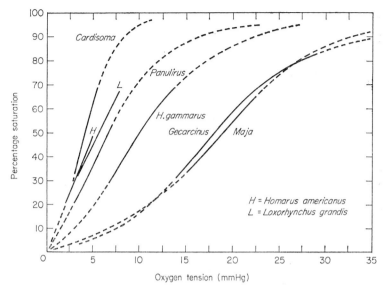

Fig. 9.5 Collected dissociation curves for bloods of decapod crustacea. The portions of the curves drawn as solid lines indicate the span between arterial and venous bloods sampled from animals in well-aerated water. (Data from authors cited in Table 9.2)

in an avoidance of oxygen-poisoning—an idea which has been explored elsewhere.[107,147]

One thing is certain; for animals living at high ambient pO_2 such a critical (or 'fail-safe') low level buffering of arterial pO_2 could only operate with an exceptionally high diffusion resistance at the respiratory organ. In the decapod crustacea this is represented by the chitinous cuticular lining of the gills which also notably limits osmotic exchanges in this group. The limitations of osmotic water influx is undoubtedly important in freshwater and estuarine forms but the limitation of arterial pO_2 in an oxygen sensitive group would be equally important in marine and terrestrial representatives such as we have been discussing. If the cuticular lining of the gill is a physiological adaptation, its role in limiting oxygen influx may be primary.

Lumbricus

In some terrestrial oligochaetes haemoglobin may be concerned in low tension transport from high external pressures but the evidence is much less complete and rather indirect. In the earthworm *Lumbricus terrestris*, the pigment has a high oxygen affinity; the following values of p_{50} have been found—at pH 7.3, 2 mm at 7° and 8 mm at 20°C[77]; at 10°C, 3.5 mm at pH 7.7 and 4.8 mm at pH 7.2.[146] Thus there is a normal temperature effect and a moderate normal Bohr effect. Such a pigment might be functional at normal atmospheric pO_2 (with large diffusion barrier at the respiratory surface as in decapods) or constitute an 'emergency' transport system which comes into play when ambient pO_2 declines. Although earthworms survive well in air-saturated water, their frequent appearance on the surface of the soil after heavy rain suggests that while water is tolerated, low ambient pO_2s are not.

Neither the sampling of arterial or venous blood nor spectroscopic examination of the blood *in vivo* has been possible and (as in the case of *Sabella*, p. 101) interpretation rests on respiration studies with the CO-method. Johnson,[104] using the method with great care, (see Fig. 9.3a p. 102) concluded that the pigment contribution varied as follows:

Ambient pO_2 (mm Hg)	152	76	38	19	8
O_2 transported by Hb ($\mu l/g/hr$)	8.0	12.3	9.8	3.4	0
% of total O_2 transported by pigment	23	35	40	22	0

It can be argued that the limiting ambient pO_2 for full arterial saturation will not be less than that at which the absolute pigment contribution begins to fall—if maximal pigment turnover can be maintained by a drop in venous pO_2 this limiting ambient level will be higher. In this case the limiting ambient pO_2 for full arterial saturation will be 76 mm or more. Since the appropriate dissociation curve[146] gives a p_{95} of c. 14 mm we can conclude that the gradient across the respiratory surface will be at least 62 mm (76–14). Such a gradient does not seem unreasonable for an animal altogether lacking specialized respiratory organs. In *Allolobophora terrestris* where the oxygen affinity of the haemoglobin is even higher than in *Lumbricus* (p_{50} is 0.7 mm at 7° and 6 mm at 20°C[77]) the diffusion barrier may be even greater.

One study has been made of a giant S. American earthworm, *Glossoscolex giganteus*, which may reach a length of 1 m and a weight of 500 g. The oxygen affinity of the haemoglobin is similar to that of *Lumbricus* ($p_{50} = 7$ mm at 20°C and pH 7.6) but the oxygen capacity is exceptionally high for an invertebrate, ranging from 10.2 to 19.8 vols % (mean 14.0). Blood obtained by catheter from the dorsal vessel was found to be 74% saturated in specimens kept in moist soil. It was argued, somewhat obscurely, that since dorsal vessel blood is a mixture of blood from the gas exchange areas and venous blood of low pO_2, a high affinity is needed, together with a very sigmoid dissociation curve, to achieve a massive oxygen turnover for a minimal further drop in pO_2.[103]

Tubifex

Superficially the situation in the aquatic oligochaete *Tubifex tubifex* is similar and this genus is sometimes linked with *Lumbricus*.[147,175] The oxygen affinity is very high (p_{50} is 0.6 mm at 17°C in the absence of CO_2[58]) and the application of the CO-method[37] indicates again that the pigment contributes substantially to oxygen uptake from air-saturation downwards (Fig. 9.3c, p. 102). However, the pattern of oxygen consumption as a function of external pO_2 shows two points of difference from that in *Lumbricus*: (a) the total and haemoglobin-less uptake is very pressure dependent over the whole pO_2 range: (b) there is a sharp break in the otherwise uniform pigment contribution at an ambient pO_2 of about 35 mm. Clearly within the range of external pO_2s studied, the demand for oxygen is insatiable; consequently, and in view of the extreme steepness of the dissociation curve, there will be little scope for maintaining the pigment contribution (when incompletely saturated) by a drop in the venous pO_2. It is probable therefore that the break in the pigment contribution curve does in this case represent the point on the ambient pO_2 scale at which the pigment ceases to be fully saturated arterially, namely 35 mm. Since p_{50} is less than 1 mm we may guess that p_{95} does not exceed 5 mm and so infer that the gradient across the unspecialized respiratory surface is of the order of 30 mm. This is a distinct improvement on the situation in *Lumbricus* and no doubt reflects a difference in the nature and role of the integument.

Since the pigment contribution is constant down to an ambient pO_2 of 35 mm, the marked pressure dependence of the total uptake must reflect other processes of uptake and distribution. Transport of oxygen in solution will be rigidly pressure dependent but the magnitude of the non-pigment mediated uptake and the steepness of this curve (Fig. 9.3) suggests that diffusion of oxygen directly to the superficial tissues without benefit of the circulatory system is also involved. It is noticeable that this 'physical' uptake curve (unlike that of pigment contribution) does not show a sharp break.

At all events, the role of *Tubifex* haemoglobin seems not to be restricted to oxygen transport from high ambient levels but in its continuing function at lower levels it provides an example to lead us on to the next section.

LOW TENSION TRANSPORT FROM LOW AMBIENT pO_2

Probably the commonest function of invertebrate respiratory pigments is the mediation of oxygen uptake via modest integumentary gradients when ambient pO_2s are low. This also requires the provision of relatively high affinity pigments but because of the small pressure drop across the respiratory surface we have the novel situation that at relatively high ambient levels the pigments remain fully saturated at the venous side of the cycle. All oxygen turned over to the tissues is then derived from the dissolved fraction of the total blood-oxygen load. Let us first examine this concept in general terms.

Concept of 'emergency' transport

In Fig. 9.6 a typical high affinity oxygen dissociation curve is shown together with the linear relationship between pO_2 and oxygen content for dissolved oxygen. In considering the yield of combined and/or dissolved oxygen, it is assumed that the metabolic needs can be met by a vols % turnover (say 0.2) which is small compared with the total blood load at full saturation. Consider first the

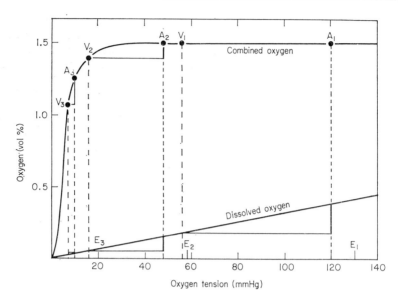

Fig. 9.6   The 'emergency' role of a high affinity respiratory pigment. With high ambient pO_2 (E_1) the required oxygen turnover comes entirely out of solution but as soon as the drop in ambient pO_2 falls below the level at which the venous tension becomes less than the loading tension, the pigment begins to contribute. This pigment contribution becomes progressively more important with further deterioration of external conditions and there is a progressive reduction in the A-V tension difference required to turnover the modest need, indicated by the thickened vertical lines, of 0.2 vols %.

situation when ambient pO_2 is E_1. With a modest gradient into arterial blood of 10 mm, arterial pO_2 and the state of the arterial pigment are represented by A_1. The fall in blood pO_2 required for a turn over of 0.2 vols % puts the venous pO_2 and the pigment state at V_1, virtually all the necessary oxygen being represented by the fall in the dissolved oxygen line. If in the absence of a pigment ambient pO_2 falls by a certain amount and the gradient across the respiratory epithelium remains the same, an undiminished turnover of dissolved oxygen can only be assured if the venous pO_2 falls by a similar amount; i.e. there is no buffering of venous pO_2 in the face of ambient reduction. Eventually ambient pO_2 might fall so low that venous pO_2 would be reduced to a level inadequate to maintain the final diffusion rate at its former level and the oxygen uptake would necessarily suffer.

If, however, the blood contains an oxygen-binding pigment the situation is radically changed. At first, a fall in ambient pO_2 will, as before, simply result in the arterial-venous cycle sliding down the pO_2 scale but a point will be reached sooner or later at which the unbuffered drop in venous pO_2 passes the loading tension of the pigment. From then on the turnover will be partly dissolved, partly combined oxygen as shown, for example, by points E_2, A_2 and V_2, in Fig. 9.6. Clearly once this point is reached venous pO_2 (but not of course arterial

pO_2) is buffered in the face of further fall in ambient pO_2. Initially this mixed contribution will include a very substantial dissolved fraction but as the A to V part of the dissociation curve becomes relatively much steeper than the dissolved oxygen line, the dissolved fraction of the total turnover may eventually become quite insignificant. At the same time the steepening of the A–V part of the curve results in A and V coming closer together—increasing buffer action and further sparing of the ultimate diffusion gradient. This very useful state of affairs is represented by points E_3, A_3 and V_3 in Fig. 9.6. Indeed the modest turnover may continue undiminished even when the ambient pO_2 falls so low that the blood is no longer fully saturated in the respiratory organ. As seen already in the decapod crustacea, an A–V difference in pO_2 of as little as 5 mm may be quite adequate even for a relatively low affinity pigment and full saturation of arterial blood is by no means essential.

The critical points in this general scheme e.g. the onset of pigment involvement and the point at which, even with the pigment, V drops so low that oxygen consumption begins to fall, are not easily defined because of the presence of other homeostatic mechanisms. We have so far assumed that circulation rate remains constant but it is probably true that this parameter is variable in most cases and helps in uptake regulation. The effect of increased circulation rate on our model would be to reduce the turnover required from a given volume of blood in order to maintain a given consumption.

Thus a high affinity pigment can be functionless at high ambient pO_2s while performing a vital function when ambient pO_2 falls below a certain level. It would thus constitute a reserve *transport facility* rather than the reserve store which many writers have postulated. Reserve storage functions cannot be entirely ruled out, as we shall see later (p. 140), but they are usually not exclusive nor even primary. In the above general account the description of external (or ambient) pO_2 as 'environmental' has been deliberately avoided, neither has the once popular expression 'emergency reserve' been used. One of the most interesting features of the role of many of these high affinity pigments is the regularity with which their reserve potential is utilized to cope not with general environmental oxygen deficiencies but with highly localized shortages often occasioned by the rhythmic nature of the animals' personal behaviour.

Chironomus and the tubicolous life

One of the best documented examples of this behavioural deprivation is found in the elegant and painstaking work of Walshe on *Chironomus*. The larvae in certain species of this genus of midges have in the haemolymph very substantial quantities of haemoglobin; they are often colloquially and very aptly called 'blood worms'. According to the most recent study of the pigment properties[221] oxygen capacity may be from 5.4 to 11.6 vols %; the dissociation curve departs only very slightly from the hyperbolic ($n = 1.1$ to 1.2); the Bohr effect though small in absolute terms is relatively large ($\Delta \log p_{50}/\Delta$ pH $= -1.04$ at 25°C; -0.54 at 15°C) and the oxygen affinity is the highest recorded (p_{50} ranges from 0.1 to 0.6

mm according to temperature and pH), apart from the problematical case of *Ascaris* and some other nematodes (p. 142).

Using the CO-method (see Fig. 9.3b), Ewer[47] demonstrated that in *C. riparius* and *C. cingulatus* normal and CO-treated larvae are capable of a similar oxygen uptake independent of pO_2 from 150 down to 60 mm. Below this point the uptake of both groups was pO_2 dependent, the uptake of CO-treated animals falling off more than that of the controls. The maximum pigment contribution appeared to occur at an ambient pO_2 of about 30 mm, being 32% of the total uptake at that level. The situation appears to illustrate very effectively our general thesis on transport from low ambient pO_2 by high (in this case very high) affinity pigments. However, since Ewer's observations were made on larvae lying free in the respirometer, we are some way from establishing the true significance of this transport function in the normal life of this tubicolous animal.

Walshe[215] began her analysis of the problem with extensive observations on the behaviour and associated state of the pigment *in vivo* for normal and CO-treated larvae housed in glass U-tubes with overlying mud and at various environmental pO_2s in the water above. With air-saturated water outside the burrow normal larvae spend on average 50% of their time in respiratory behaviour—intermittent short bursts of irrigation activity separated by pauses of up to 30 min. Actual irrigating time is limited to about 3%. Filter feeding—a very energetic series of cycles of net spinning, violent irrigation and net eating—occupied about 35% of the time; complete and prolonged immobility occupied the remaining 15%. As external (outside the burrow) pO_2 fell below 45 mm, respiratory behaviour increased, with relatively more irrigation time, and filter feeding decreased. CO-treated larvae, on the other hand, show less filter feeding (22%) even at the highest external pO_2s and this activity fell off more severely at lower levels; respiratory behaviour failed to show a compensatory increase but fell markedly below air-saturation (Fig. 9.7). The limiting external pO_2 for filter feeding was 15 mm in normal larvae but 40 mm in CO-treated ones. The rate of recovery from the complete immobility induced by anoxia was in all cases proportional to the pO_2 of water above the burrow but while the limiting pO_2 for such recovery was 11 mm for normal animals it was 23 mm for treated ones. The advantage of the pigment is clear when environmental pO_2 is low but it remains to be seen whether use is restricted to such periods and what is its precise nature.

The blood-worm particularly lends itself to spectroscopic examination of the pigment *in vivo* and although arterial and venous blood cannot be distinguished, the composite picture of the overall pigment state can give some useful indications. If complete oxygenation of the pigment is seen only the dissolved fraction of the blood oxygen is being used; if partial deoxygenation is apparent some effective turnover of combined oxygen is indicated; complete deoxygenation indicates complete anoxia.

Walshe found that with air-saturated water available larvae spent only 3% of their time actually irrigating and as a consequence, for 21% of the animals' time partial deoxygenation indicated effective transport by the pigment, while during the latter part of the frequent irrigation pauses complete deoxygenation of the

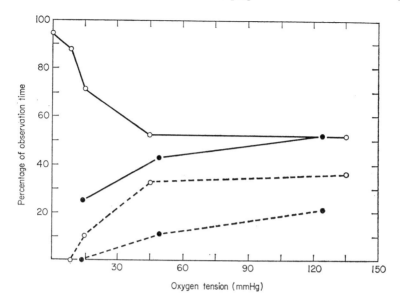

Fig. 9.7 Variations in the behaviour of larvae of *Chironomus plumosus* with changing pO_2 in the water overlying the burrow. ——— respiratory behaviour, - - - - - filter feeding; o normal animals, ● CO-treated animals. (From Walshe[215])

pigment prevails (41%). With an external pO_2 of only 23–15 mm active irrigation occupies 50% of the time and dissolved oxygen is adequate for 45% while the periods of pigment transport and complete anaerobiosis fall to 27 and 28% respectively. For air-saturation conditions complete deoxygenation of the pigment takes 19 min from the beginning of the irrigation pause, a period which must represent the transport of residual oxygen in the burrow water plus the storage value of the pigment. With a low external pO_2 of 23–15 mm complete oxygenation prevails so long as irrigation is uninterrupted but deoxygenation is complete 9 min from the beginning of the pause. This figure must represent approximately the storage potential of the pigment since under these conditions the residual oxygen in the burrow would be very little. At the end of the pause, 1.5 min of continuous irrigation with well-aerated water suffices to restore the pigment to full oxygenation when the next pause begins. At the low external pO_2, 6 min irrigation is required to recharge the pigment and a further 4 min activity precedes the next pause.

Animals rendered apnoeic by artificial irrigation of the burrow with well-aerated water, can be taken through the deoxygenation/reoxygenation cycle passively, without themselves pursuing any irrigation activity and with water of varying pO_2 to induce recovery. Reoxygenation is always faster and deoxygenation always slower than for normally active animals at similar pO_2s—an indication of the cost of irrigation and other muscular activity.

Obviously, the precise role of the haemoglobin is complex. So long as water with a pO_2 in excess of about 15 mm is passing over the body the pigment remains fully saturated and the animal's needs are satisfied by dissolved oxygen in the blood. But since the animal never spends all its time irrigating, the pigment assumes a role with every irrigation pause, even with air-saturated water above the mud. The haemoglobin firstly expedites transport of residual oxygen in the burrow, secondly acts as a store for a short time (probably about 9 min) and finally facilitates recovery from the anaerobiosis of the latter part of the pause. Furthermore, filter feeding, which is a very energetic process and apparently an essentially aerobic one, can only be fully sustained at any particular environmental pO_2 by virtue of the pigment. Here the role is probably one of maintaining fully aerobic internal conditions during mucus secretion and spinning when irrigation is necessarily suspended.

A most interesting feature of these findings is that in addition to its importance, especially in facilitating feeding, at low environmental pO_2, the pigment is constantly being utilized in 'emergencies' which are of the animal's own making and a consequence of its rhythmic way of life. Such rhythmic or cyclic patterns with consequential local (or strictly ambient) oxygen deficiencies must be a common feature of tubicolous life (e.g. *Arenicola*, the sipunculids) and this kind of pigment role is probably fairly common. Although many examples have been carefully described and analysed as to controlling factors, we lack studies of the 'economics' of activity cycles in tubicolous forms. In *Chironomus* and in others it is not simply that irrigation activity must of necessity give way periodically to some other vital but incompatible activity, such as feeding. It seems highly probable that a regulated cycle of aerobic and anaerobic phases provides a useful compromise between the energy/food economy of aerobiosis and the high metabolic cost of irrigation by muscular action—it is notable that irrigation of a tube or burrow by ciliary action is not regularly intermittent.

Walshe's later studies[217] shed an interesting light on another aspect of the tubicolous habit in *Chironomus*. She determined the relationship of oxygen consumption to pO_2 in all possible combinations of the following circumstances: larvae in tubes and without tubes; with and without functional haemoglobin; adapted (by overnight exposure to the pO_2 of the ensuing experiment) and non-adapted. A summary of the results is given in Fig. 9.8.

The difference between tubeless, non-adapted larvae with and without haemoglobin (Fig. 9.8b) agreed well with Ewer's original observations (Fig. 9.3b, p. 102) but these were the least natural circumstances. Prior adaptation of tubeless larvae made virtually no difference in either CO-treated or normal larvae; uptake remained markedly pressure dependent in both groups and significant pigment contribution still occurred apparently only below 65 mm (Fig. 9.8a). Non-adapted larvae in tubes showed the most pronounced pressure dependence over the whole range, with pigment contribution apparent only below 38 mm (Fig. 9.8d). In the most natural conditions, adapted larvae in tubes were less pressure dependent than those in any other circumstances but the pigment contribution was still only significant below 65 mm (Fig. 9.8c). The greatest difference of

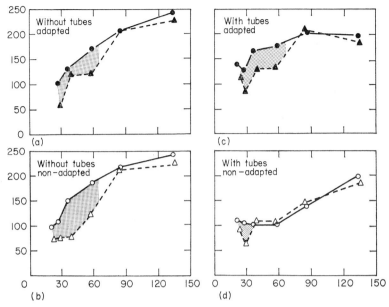

Fig. 9.8 Oxygen consumption of larvae of *Chironomus plumosus* as a function of dissolved oxygen tension under various conditions. Co-ordinates to common scales—ordinate: oxygen consumption in $\mu l/g/hr$; abscissa: pO_2 in mm Hg. Continuous lines—normal animals; broken lines—CO-treated animals; stippled areas—range of significant differences. (After Walshe-Maetz[217])

all occurred between adapted and non-adapted larvae in tubes and with haemoglobin (solid lines in Figs. 9.8c and d), the adapted larvae taking up more oxygen at all tensions below 95 mm. Adaptation is therefore a most important but essentially tubicolous feature and is probably concerned with the manner of response to the accumulation of acid metabolites by irrigation.

Finally, a comparative re-examination was made of the behaviour of two subspecies—*C. plumosus plumosus* and *C. plumosus flaveolus*. In the former (subject of the above-mentioned oxygen uptake experiments) irrigation pauses were so short, even at higher pO_2s outside the burrow, that the pigment never became even partially deoxygenated during the pauses—so the pigment role is limited to periods of true environmental oxygen deficiency, of feeding and of prolonged immobility. In *C. p. flaveolus*, on the other hand (subject of the original behaviour studies), the relative 'laziness' was confirmed along with the consequent periods of partial and complete deoxygenation. In the latter subspecies, however, CO-treated animals tended to compensate by increased irrigation activity—a factor which would tend to mask the normal/CO difference in oxygen uptake measurements and reduce the validity of the carbon monoxide method.

These studies by Walshe provide a classic demonstration of two points of great general importance, namely the need for a thorough understanding of the animal's way of life and for measuring physiological parameters under conditions resembling as closely as possible those of the natural environment. These generalities are further illustrated by our next example.

Aquatic pulmonates—*Planorbis* and *Lymnaea*

The respiration of aquatic pulmonate gastropods is potentially interesting for two related reasons. These animals are secondarily aquatic and for the most part have retained the well-vascularized mantle in its former terrestrial role as a lung. Accordingly, in these forms, the exchange of oxygen and carbon dioxide is potentially possible with both air and water. Work on the respiratory pigments in such forms has largely concentrated on *Planorbis corneus** (the familiar ramshorn) simply because of the conspicuously high haemoglobin concentration in its blood. Many early writers on invertebrate respiratory pigments (e.g. Leitch,[136] Borden[21]) asserted, usually referring to *Planorbis* among others, that 'the presence of haemoglobin in the invertebrates has generally been found to be correlated with a *habitat* at times deficient in oxygen' (my italics). Much early and also more recent work has tended to pre-judge this issue, taking the deficiencies of the environment for granted, and set out to show how the pigment may help to sustain aerobic metabolism in difficult circumstances by detailed study of the properties *in vitro*.

Planorbis haemoglobin has a fairly high oxygen affinity (p_{50} at 20°C lies in the region 3 to 7 mm for the probable physiological range of pH) and has a moderate negative (normal) Bohr effect[237] in the physiological range. The oxygen capacity of the blood is rather variable but values up to 2.5 vols % have been recorded.[108] There is again little doubt that this pigment is potentially very useful for low tension oxygen transport but, as with *Chironomus*, more information is required to establish the full nature of its biological role. Some attempts to elucidate the broader respiratory picture were made by Jordan,[112] Probst[171] and Füsser and Krüger[65] but did not seem to be conclusive. A further effort was made[106] to relate the known properties of the pigment to overall respiratory performance and the actual life of the animal. Partly in order to avoid dependence on the CO-method, a parallel study was made on *Lymnaea stagnalis* (another pulmonate often found living alongside *Planorbis corneus*) which was widely thought to lack a respiratory pigment, acting as a form of control. The parallel study proved unexpectedly useful.

In both these species the snails forage below the surface but periodically and even in well-aerated water, crawl to the surface and open the pulmonary cavity to the air via a narrow aperture for a period of up to 1 or even 2 minutes. Diffusion exchange of gases occurs and there is no mechanical ventilation. The ensuing

---

* This animal should strictly be referred to the genus *Planorbarius* but in the present context I am reluctant to change the name by which it has been known to students of respiratory pigments for a century—Ray Lankester identified the red pigment as a haemoglobin in 1869.[132]

dive is variable but may last up to two hours or more if the animal finds difficulty in regaining the surface. Several observers have suggested that the duration of the dive is longer in *Planorbis* than in *Lymnaea*. It was found that in shallow water with abundant vegetation (such as *Elodea, Cladophora, Phragmites* etc.) reaching the surface, *Planorbis* had a marked tendency to forage on the bottom-mud using the plants mainly as a means of access to the surface, while *Lymnaea* tended to browse on the plants and consequently always had 'a foot on the ladder' when the need arose to return to the surface.

The detailed comparative study was made on a mixed population in a typical Dutch polderland ditch near Leiden; the limpid water was only 15 to 20 cm deep and in summer the vegetation filled and eventually choked the ditch. Dissolved oxygen tensions in the upper layers exhibit a remarkable diurnal cycle in such conditions due to the photosynthesis. On a sunny day in June values ranged from 10 mm pO_2 at 03.30 hrs to 490 mm at 13.30 hrs, with conditions of super-saturation (> 150 mm) for about 14 hours at a stretch (Fig. 4.1, p. 20). The pO_2 increase is of course partly due to rise in temperature. Close to the bottom the corresponding extremes were 10 and 100 mm. Earlier in the season maxima were less extreme because of lower temperatures and because the thinner vegetation permitted effective vertical mixing; in May diurnal maxima for bottom and upper layers were similar at about 300 mm (still twice saturation). Maximum pCO_2 determined just before sunrise was about 15 mm in June.

In aquaria, dive durations are not significantly different in the two species because both have equally easy access to the surface and, since the stimulus to return is at least partly due to loss of buoyancy in the shell, starting off at similar times in search of the surface are likely to arrive after a similar interval. However, the duration of the dive is clearly directly related to dissolved pO_2. When total pulmonary and cutaneous oxygen uptake for the duration of simulated dives were determined separately but simultaneously for both species an interesting contrast was found (Figs. 9.9 and 9.10). In each species cutaneous uptake declines with fall in dissolved oxygen tension and this is accompanied by a compensatory rise in uptake from the lung, so that total uptake is constant over a wide ambient range. Hence the pulmonary oxygen reserve is more rapidly depleted and the dive duration shortened. However, in spite of its lack of respiratory pigment *Lymnaea* sustains during its shorter dive a higher total uptake than *Planorbis* at all dissolved tensions but is more dependent on its lung. Pulmonary uptake exceeds cutaneous at all dissolved tensions below 160 mm in *Lymnaea* but only below 100 mm in *Planorbis*. In these experiments the simulated dive allowed *Lymnaea* to refill its lung twice as frequently as *Planorbis* so it was to be expected that the mean pulmonary pO_2 would be higher in the former—as is shown below this is true in natural dives. It appears therefore that the lung performs a sort of 'topping-up' function and pulmonary oxygen is spared when pO_2 in the water is high. The arrangement of the vascular system determines this because, whilst only part of the venous blood passes through cutaneous sinuses and is open to oxygena-tion via the skin, all blood (except for the renal supply) is subsequently pooled and passes through the pulmonary capillary bed on its way back to the heart.

When measurements were made of pulmonary gas composition at the beginning and end of natural dives in the ditch, it was found that in neither case did the lung contents equilibrate fully with the atmosphere during lung-opening. Initial pulmonary pO_2 averaged 120 mm in *Planorbis* and 135 mm in *Lymnaea* but the difference was not significant. At the end of the dive there is a highly significant difference (both statistically and biologically), final pulmonary pO_2 for *Planorbis* being 21 mm, for *Lymnaea* 65 mm (Table 9.3). Knowing the initial volume of

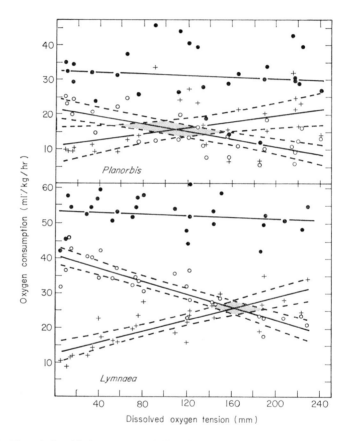

Fig. 9.9 The relationship between total (•), pulmonary (o) and cutaneous (+) oxygen uptake and the dissolved oxygen tension in the water for *Planorbis corneus* and *Lymnaea stagnalis*. The solid lines represent the regressions of oxygen uptake on pO_2, the broken lines indicate 95% confidence limits and the shaded areas show the pO_2 ranges in which pulmonary and cutaneous uptake are practically equal. The slopes of the total uptake regression lines are not significantly different from the horizontal, i.e. total uptake is constant. The distinction between the two species in respect of absolute oxygen uptake values is exaggerated by plotting results on a total weight basis; on a tissue weight basis there is a smaller difference—see Fig. 9.10 where the picture is much clearer. (Jones[106])

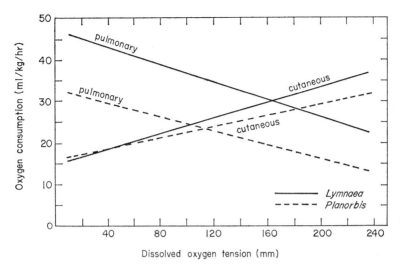

Fig. 9.10 The regression lines for pulmonary and cutaneous oxygen uptake from Fig. 9.9, recalculated on a tissue weight basis to allow for the difference in relative weight of the shell in the two species.

pulmonary gas per g of tissue weight* and the change during the dive, it was possible to calculate the utilization of the pulmonary oxygen during the dive;[108] that for *Planorbis* (0.044 ml/g) is about twice that for *Lymnaea* (0.021 ml/g) (Table 9.4).

It is interesting that in neither species is there a significant accumulation of carbon dioxide in the lung during the dive (Table 9.3). This is not surprising for aquatic animals in a medium with a low ambient (dissolved) pCO_2. This gas diffuses so readily across the epithelium of all exposed surfaces into a medium in which it is highly soluble, that only a very slight gradient is needed for cutaneous elimination.

The tentative conclusions to be drawn at this stage are : (a) whatever the role of the pigment in *Planorbis vis-à-vis* cutaneous uptake when dissolved pO_2 is low, the pulmonary pressure falls to such a low level during the latter part of the normal dive that dissolved oxygen transport is then likely to prove inadequate and the relatively high affinity pigment will be called into play to permit maximal exploitation of the pulmonary gas; (b) when lacking a pigment *Lymnaea* is unable to exploit the lower part of its pulmonary oxygen store but can nevertheless maintain an equal (if not slightly higher) rate of aerobic metabolism by coming to the surface more frequently to renew its pulmonary reserve; (c) this difference governs the difference in foraging behaviour and as a consequence the two species occupy different ecological niches within the same habitat.

* Comparisons on a tissue weight basis are more meaningful because the shell accounts for 32% of total weight in *Planorbis*, only 14% in *Lymnaea*.

This hypothesis would be strengthened if it could be shown that the lower level of pulmonary pO_2, below the point where *Lymnaea* gives up, does correspond to the region in which *Planorbis* haemoglobin is actively contributing. An attempt was made to test this in the most direct manner by spectroscopic examination of the pigment *in vivo* using the albino variety which lacks cutaneous melanin.[108] Points were chosen where, with certain precautions and reservations, distinctive views could be obtained of blood before and after passing the pulmonary circulation (venous and arterial blood).

The animal, fixed on its side inside a small Perspex chamber (Fig. 9.11), could be perfused with water of varying pO_2 and was encouraged to adopt a normal posture and activity by being provided with a treadmill. The following observations were made with oxygen-free water. Viewing arterial blood in the pulmonary vein with the spectroscope, the animal was quickly released and the pulmonary gas sampled as soon as the blood just ceased to show any signs of oxygenation. This lower limit of pulmonary oxygen for zero saturation of arterial blood would set the lower limit on usefulness of the pigment and the remaining pO_2 in the lung would approximate to the pulmonary gradient, arterial pO_2 being close to zero. The values obtained for this limit were between 15 and 20 mm. Similarly,

Table 9.3 Pulmonary gas composition in natural dives. Oxygen and carbon dioxide percentages and partial pressures (mmHg) in the lung at the beginning and the end of dives in the natural habitat (described in the text) for three aquatic pulmonates. For oxygen the initial percentages are not significantly different between species, neither are final percentages as between *Planorbis* and *Biomphalaria*. Significant accumulation of carbon dioxide during the dive occurs only in *Biomphalaria*. (Jones[109])

		Lymnaea		*Planorbis*		*Biomphalaria*	
		p.p.	%	p.p.	%	p.p	%
O_2	Initial	135	18.2	120	16.2	109*	17.1
	Final	65	8.8	21	2.8	19	2.9
CO_2	Initial	8	1.1	9	1.2	11	1.7
	Final	8	1.1	10	1.3	16	2.5

* Barometric pressure in the region of Lake Victoria is only 660 mm.

Table 9.4 Utilization of pulmonary oxygen during the dive—calculated on the basis of tissue weight. (Jones[109])

		Lymnaea	*Planorbis*	*Biomphalaria*
Initial pulmonary gas vol (ml/g)		0.20	0.32	0.36
Change during the dive	% O_2	9.4	13.4	14.2
	mm pO_2	70.0	99.2	90.5*
Utilized O_2 vol (ml/g)		0.021	0.044	0.045

* Barometric pressure in the region of Lake Victoria is only 660 mm.

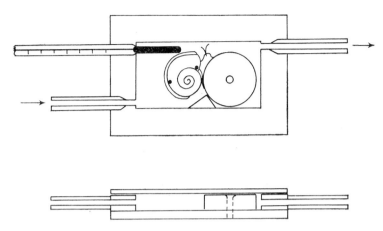

Fig. 9.11 Perfusion/observation chamber for use on the microscope stage to study the *in vitro* state of the haemoglobin of *Planorbis* and its relation to changing pO_2 in the external water or in pulmonary gas. The black spots indicate the arterial and venous viewpoints referred to in the description of the method in the text. (Jones[108])

viewing blood in the circulus venosus, the limiting pulmonary pO_2 was determined at which this venous blood just began to depart from 100% saturation—this value was about 50 to 60 mm. At higher values the pigment must be fully oxygenated throughout the circulation and all turnover be derived from dissolved oxygen. Despite the rather crude method of determination, there is a very satisfactory agreement between these limits and the lower pulmonary limits determined at the end of natural dives in *Planorbis* and *Lymnaea* respectively (Table 9.3).

Subsequently, the opportunity occurred to make some observations on another haemoglobin-bearing planorbid, *Biomphalaria sudanica*, living in the completely anoxic waters of the papyrus swamps in Uganda.[109] Data for this species are also included in Tables 9.3 and 9.4. In all important respects *Biomphalaria* closely resembles *Planorbis* and so differs from *Lymnaea* in the same significant way. It would appear that *Planorbis* is so well adapted to the task of maximal exploitation of pulmonary oxygen that there is no room for improvement in the even more adverse respiratory conditions encountered by *Biomphalaria*. One possibly significant difference between the two planorbids is illustrated in Fig. 9.12. If allowance is made for the different temperatures and carbon dioxide tensions of the respective environments, the probable functional dissociation curves (a and b) are very similar although in absolute terms *Planorbis* haemoglobin has an appreciably lower oxygen affinity and would be less well suited to life at the high temperature and pCO_2 of the swamp waters.

In the initial studies on the Dutch polderland *Lymnaea*, it was found that there were traces of copper in the blood (up to 2 ppm) which, if representing haemocyanin, would contribute an oxygen capacity of only 0.04 vols %—a scarcely

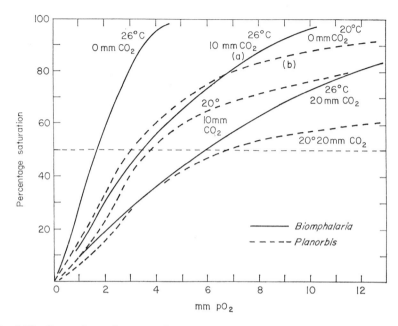

mm pO_2

Fig. 9.12 Comparison of oxygen dissociation curves of whole blood of *Biomphalaria sudanica* and *Planorbis corneus* equilibrated with 0, 10 and 20 mm pCO_2 at standard environmental temperatures. (See discussion in the text.) (Jones[109]; data for *Planorbis* from Zaaijer and Wolvekamp[237])

significant amount. Later studies on *Lymnaea stagnalis* in Yorkshire[110] have revealed a somewhat different situation which nevertheless seems to confirm the original interpretations. Only one out of seven populations examined in the Sheffield area contained snails whose blood was consistently colourless and even these contained more copper than the Dutch snails (4 to 6.5 ppm Cu—means of large samples taken periodically over two years). Sample means for the other populations ranged from 7 to 22 ppm. The highest individual value ever recorded was 49 ppm and although even this maximal figure only represents an oxygen capacity of 0.86 vols %, there are reasons for thinking that in these 'high copper' snails the pigment comes to assume a significant oxygen transport function and that this is similar to that already suggested for *Planorbis*.

The magnitude of the copper titre could not be correlated with differences in the prevailing dissolved oxygen tension but the 'low copper' snails did enjoy one distinctive physical feature. Their pond resembled the Dutch ditches in that the water was shallow and supported an abundance of aquatic plants whose stems reached the surface or beyond it, thus providing an extensive feeding area with direct access to the surface. All the 'high copper' snails were found in larger ponds virtually devoid of any but encrusting vegetation and with margins shelving more or less steeply down to considerable depths. In these circumstances foraging often took the snails long distances from the edge and the surface could only be regained by a long crawl up the shore. Detailed study in the native habitats of dive duration and final composition of the pulmonary gas showed that while the 'low copper' snails behaved essentially like those in the Dutch ditches, the performance of the 'high copper' individuals much more resembled that of the Dutch *Planorbis* (Table 9.5).

Table 9.5 Respiratory performance—diving in the natural habitat (for explanation see text). (Jones[110])

Locality	Leiden	*Lymnaea* Woodsetts (low Cu)	Wintersett (high Cu)	*Planorbis* Leiden
Final pulmonary pO_2 (mm)	65	76	20	21
Duration of dive (min)	*c.* 30?	38	90	60
Blood copper (ppm)	3	3.9	11.6	—
Water pO_2 (mm)	up to 400	up to 206	up to 226	up to 400

In an attempt to test the obvious deduction, snails from each population were transferred to a small artificial pond which, in respect of lack of vegetation and more difficult access to the surface, more closely resembled the natural habitat of the 'high copper' snails. Their respective performances were compared with those of a population of *Planorbis* which had established itself apparently by natural means in the artificial pond. In view of the very marked adaptation which occurred in the copper content of the 'low copper' snails over a period of 10 weeks, a further batch of these were transferred and their performance measured in the new habitat after only two days. The data from these transfer experiments are summarized in Table 9.6. It is curious that all the *Lymnaea* in the artificial

Table 9.6 Respiratory performance on transfer to artificial pond (for explanation see text). (Jones[110])

Origin and adaptation	Wintersett adapted	*Lymnaea* Woodsetts adapted	Woodsetts non-adapted	*Planorbis* 'native'
Final pulmonary pO_2 (mm)	44	41	43	21
Duration of dive (min)	51	53	108	112
Blood copper (ppm)	18.1	15.3	5.7	—

pond finished their dives with the same oxygen content. The 'high copper' snails evidently found it easier to get back to the surface here than in their native pond, for they had about twice as much oxygen left but had been submerged only about half as long (cf. Table 9.5). The non-adapted 'low copper' snails found difficulty in regaining the surface, making dives of over 100 min but even in this time did not get the final percentage of O_2 much below 6%—the latter parts of these dives were probably fairly anaerobic. On the other hand, given a period of

E

acclimatization, there was a striking threefold increase in copper content of the blood (confirmed by a similar rise in the second batch of transferred 'low copper' snails) and a possibly learned shortening of the dive. The shorter dives terminated with about the same pulmonary oxygen level as before but must have been much less anaerobic. Meanwhile the *Planorbis* were putting up a typical performance with a final pulmonary pO_2 of 21 mm after 112 min.

If under the stimulus of adverse respiratory conditions (more difficult access to the surface) *Lymnaea* can respond by imitating *Planorbis*, does the increasing quantity of respiratory pigment have similar properties? Fig. 9.13 shows that in respect of oxygen affinity it does. The dissociation curve of *Lymnaea* haemocyanin is much more like that of *Planorbis* haemoglobin than that of *Helix* haemocyanin.

As in the case of *Chironomus*, the role of the pigment is related primarily to alleviating the consequences of oxygen deprivation due not to simple environmental deficiency but to behavioural consequences. *Lymnaea* illustrates both sides of the coin; so long as the nature of the habitat permits short dives no oxygen transport pigment is needed but when longer dives become necessary a haemocyanin with appropriate properties can be synthesized.

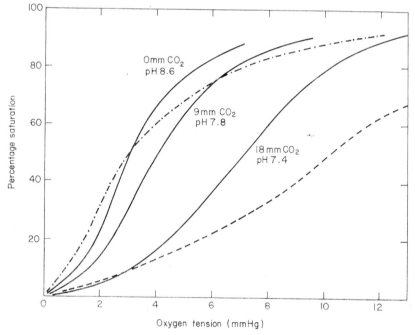

Fig. 9.13   Oxygen dissociation curves of whole blood of *Lymnaea stagnalis* at 15 °C and various pCO_2s, showing a fairly high oxygen affinity and a normal Bohr effect. The other curves are for *Planorbis* blood (-·-·-·-·) at 20 °C and 0 mm pCO_2 and for *Helix* blood (------) at 15 °C and 0 mm pCO_2. (*Planorbis* curve from Zaaijer and Wolvekamp[237]; *Helix* curve from Spoek et al[204])

SIGNIFICANCE OF VARIATIONS IN THE BOHR EFFECT

Magnitude of the Bohr effect

In some of the examples discussed above there may be a marginal advantage in the normal Bohr effect which the respective pigments have been shown to possess. Such an advantage would lie in steepening of the functional dissociation curve when account is taken of the difference in pCO_2 between arterial and venous blood (see p. 99). So far as the potentialities of the pigment itself are concerned, it is possible to express the magnitude of the Bohr effect numerically as the shift in P_{50} per unit change in pH or $\Delta \log p_{50}/\Delta$ pH; some examples estimated for the physiological range of pH are given in Table 9.7. The value of this ratio is not constant in a particular species, as is apparent from a consideration of Fig. 8.5, nor does it indicate by itself the significance of the Bohr effect since it does not

Table 9.7 Magnitude of the Bohr effect expressed as $\Delta \log.p_{50}/\Delta pH$. All the vertebrate values are for haemoglobin solutions except those in brackets which are for whole blood. Values for mammalian Hb solutions from Riggs;[185] for whole blood from Bartels;[13] for the remainder see the authors indicated. Values for *Loligo* and *Busycon* have been roughly estimated from the data of the original authors.

White mouse	-0.96	(-0.61)	Mackerel[175]	-1.2
Guinea pig	-0.79	(-0.47)		
Rabbit	-0.75	(-0.45)	*Petromyzon*[148]	-0.7
Dog	-0.65	(-0.50)	*Polistotrema*[148]	0.0
Man	-0.62	(-0.50)		
Pig	-0.57	(-0.42)	*Eupolymnia*[146]	0.0
Cow	-0.52	(-0.49)	*Spirographis*[175]	-0.66
Elephant	-0.38	(-0.37)	*Lumbricus*[175]	-0.25
			Loligo[178]	-1.8
Bullfrog adult[184]	-0.24		*Busycon*[176]	$+0.2$
Bullfrog tadpole	0.0		*Fasciolaria*[182]	$+1.26$
			Fusitriton[182]	$+2.12$

take into account the actual A-V pCO_2 difference or the pH change which occurs when this increased carbon dioxide is buffered (see p. 168). Only when all the relevant respiratory parameters are known can the functional significance be fully established. In a resting man, blood pCO_2 increases from 40 to 47 mm but the plasma pH falls only by about 0.03 units (7.43–7.40), sufficient to reduce the saturation of the venous blood from 75 (in the absence of the Bohr effect) to 74%. With an arterial saturation of 95%, this represents a 5% improvement in the oxygen turnover. At work, the accumulation of lactic acid in the blood may lower the pH of arterial blood but the increased carbon dioxide load will also increase the A-V pH difference. With a difference of 0.07 units (7.35–7.28) when metabolic rate is $7 \times$ basal, the venous pO_2 falls to about 31 mm (cf. 40 mm at rest) and the venous saturation is about 50%. In the absence of the Bohr effect a venous saturation of 56% would be found, hence in this case the improvement in turnover is 6/39 or about 15%.[20] This does not represent the limit of advantage since considerably larger A-V pH differences are found within physiological limits. Further, the exercise example given probably underestimates the advantage, since the venous parameters are based on samples of mixed venous blood and may not fully reflect the changes in the active tissues.

A moderate inverse correlation has been found between the magnitude of the Bohr effect and body weight in mammals, the value of the ratio $\Delta \log p_{50}/\Delta pH$ ranging from -0.38 in the elephant to -0.6 in the shrew. There is also a similar inverse correlation for p_{50}, so that a change in blood pH from 7.4 to 7.2 raises p_{50} from 37 to 49 mm in the shrew and from 22 to 26 mm in the elephant.[13] Taking these two factors together there is, therefore, a neat adjustment of facility for unloading to match the intensity of metabolism.*

In aquatic animals generally there is a tendency for blood pCO_2 and the A-V difference to be low because of the relative ease with which this gas can diffuse out of the body by a variety of routes. Even in the decapod crustacea, with their well-developed external skeletons, the differences are usually less than 1 mm and the corresponding pH changes less than 0.1 unit (see Table 9.2, p. 105). In these circumstances the Bohr effect is of little consequence.

Role of the Bohr effect in the squid

A notable exception among aquatic invertebrates is the American squid *Loligo pealei* whose haemocyanin is exceptionally sensitive to pH change, $\Delta \log p_{50}/\Delta pH$ being about -1.8. This low affinity pigment provides a good example of high tension transport in an invertebrate; it also illustrates *par excellence* the functional advantage of the normal (negative) Bohr effect. Redfield and Goodkind[178] made one of the earliest invertebrate studies involving measurement of the important respiratory parameters of both arterial and venous blood. For animals in air-saturated water arterial blood contained a total of 4.27 vols % oxygen at a tension of 120 mm and 3.98 vols % carbon dioxide at a tension of 2 mm, while venous blood contained 0.37 vols % ($\equiv 48$ mm) and 8.27 vols % ($\equiv 6$ mm) respectively. The 4 mm difference in pCO_2 corresponds to a pH change of 0.13 units.

Taken together with earlier studies of the oxygen equilibrium of the pigment,[176] these data yield the picture given in Fig. 9.14. In a total oxygen turnover of 3.9 vols % the pigment is responsible for about 3.75 vols % and about 37% of this is due to the change in pCO_2. A Bohr effect of this magnitude carries with it the danger that an increase in ambient pCO_2 (and hence of arterial pCO_2) will seriously reduce the oxygen saturation of arterial blood. In an animal which evidently depends on a relatively complete turnover of its combined oxygen, this is likely to have grave consequences. Indeed, Redfield and Goodkind were able to demonstrate this practically by determining the lethal low level of pO_2 at various ambient pCO_2s. With an ambient pCO_2 of 1 mm squids survived until

* Two other related parameters appear to be inversely correlated with body weight in mammals: (a) the extent of increase of p_{50} by carbon dioxide *at constant pH*;[185] (b) the concentration of carbonic anhydrase in the erythrocytes.[133]

pO_2 fell to between 20 and 35 mm, while with a pCO_2 of 20 mm the critical pO_2 rose to about 100 mm.

The massive turnover of 86% of combined oxygen in the relatively inactive experimental animals (they were restrained with forced ventilation during sampling procedures) raises a problem, as yet unresolved. It was estimated that the circulation rate in the restrained squids was about 11 ml/kg body wt/min. Taken

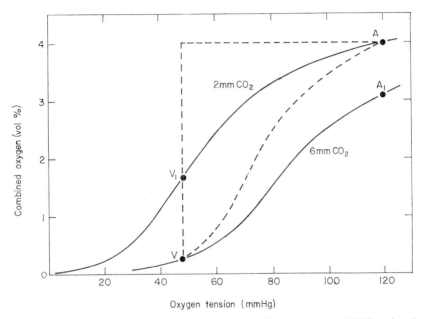

Oxygen tension (mmHg)

Fig. 9.14 Oxygen dissociation curves for the blood of *Loligo pealei* at 23 °C and at the pCO_2 of arterial and venous blood respectively. Points A and V represent the conditions in arterial and venous blood for animals in well-aerated water which is virtually CO_2-free. The line V-V_1 indicates the increase in oxygen turnover which is due to the very pronounced negative Bohr effect. A_1 represents the condition which would be found in arterial blood if the ambient pCO_2 were to rise by as little as 4 mm ; the saturation defiency could not be made good however low venous pO_2 were to fall. (Drawn from the data of Redfield and Goodkind[178])

with the total oxygen turn over of 3.9 vols %, this would yield only about 0.43 ml/kg/min or 26 ml/kg/hr, compared with a measured oxygen consumption of about 600 ml/kg/hr in actively swimming animals. Since the venous blood is only 8% saturated (cf. over 70% in a resting man) we cannot look to an increase in the respiratory turnover for provision of the oxygen needs at high and continuous levels of swimming activity. It must be presumed that there is a massive increase in circulatory rate but this would put a high premium on the efficiency of transfer across the gill epithelium. It is known that utilization of oxygen (p. 15) may reach the unusually high level of 80% in *Octopus* so there may well be in this group scope for respiratory regulation along these lines. Clearly the relationships between rates of oxygen consumption, circulation, ventilation and utilization merit further study.

It appears that the squid is endowed with a respiratory system capable of sustaining a very high level of activity only by exploiting to the full at all times the advantages of its unusual blood pigment. There is little in reserve to meet the problems of externally lowered oxygen or increased carbon dioxide tensions but these problems will not be met by a pelagic marine animal.

Other cephalopods

The magnitude of the Bohr effect is less in other cephalopod groups and probably for good functional reasons. While the data for representative cuttlefishes and octopuses are much less complete, Wolvekamp[231] has suggested that the differences which are known reflect differences in habitat and activity. Squids are active pelagic animals, while cuttlefishes (such as *Sepia*) mostly swim rather slowly at lower levels or lie in wait for their prey on the sea-bed and octopuses crawl over the bottom and spend much time concealed in holes or crevices. This sequence is paralleled by a marked tendency for an increase in the oxygen affinity and a decrease in the Bohr effect of the respective haemocyanins. These trends should lend the non-pelagic forms a progressively greater tolerance of lowered pO_2 and raised pCO_2 in the external medium, though at the expense of the capacity for very high levels of activity. This is an attractive hypothesis which calls for experimental analysis.

Aquatic vertebrates

In many aquatic animals the Bohr effect is absent and in some of these one may confidently postulate that this situation is a positive adaptation to special living conditions. Thus, in the bullfrog *Rana catesbeiana* the tadpole haemoglobin is quite insensitive to pCO_2, while the adult pigment shows a moderate negative Bohr effect ($\Delta\log p_{50}/\Delta pH = -0.24$) (Fig. 8.5 p. 91). This development is thought to reflect the change from a crowded and stagnant aquatic habitat subject to great variation in pO_2 and pCO_2, where the loading disadvantages of a Bohr effect would far outweigh the unloading advantages, to an air-breathing habit ensuring a consistently low ambient pCO_2 and high pO_2. At the same time there is a marked lowering of oxygen affinity (p_{50} increases from 4 to about 25 mm).

The data for the bullfrog quoted above were obtained from haemoglobin solutions and must therefore be viewed with caution. However, striking differences have also been found between the whole blood properties for 'larval' and 'adult' axolotls (*Ambystoma mexicanum*). Following artificially induced metamorphosis there is a fourfold increase in metabolic rate and a 40% drop in weight. This is paralleled by a slight fall in oxygen affinity ($p_{50} = 26$ to 29 mm), a marked increase in the sigmoidness of the dissociation curve ($n = 2$ to 3.4) and a very significant increase in the Bohr effect ($\Delta\log p_{50}/\Delta pH$ -0.14 to -0.26).[66]

A similar contrast is found in cyclostomes between adult hagfish and lampreys. In the former, respiratory conditions are adverse with low ambient pO_2 and variable pCO_2 because of the habit of burrowing either into the bodies of dead or dying fish or in mud. The problem is met by oxygen transport at low tension and in the complete (*Polistotrema*) or virtual (*Myxine*) absence of a Bohr effect. The ectoparasitic sea lamprey *Petromyzon marinus*, on the other hand, is assured of a continuous supply of well-aerated water at consistently low pCO_2; accordingly it makes good use of a low affinity haemoglobin with a pronounced Bohr effect.[148] Considerations of a like nature seem to govern variations in carbon dioxide sensitivity among teleost fishes. Sluggish or stagnant water forms tend to show small Bohr effects, while inhabitants of fast-moving water and very active species show large responses to small changes in pCO_2 (in the mackerel $\Delta \log p_{50}/\Delta pH$ is -1.2).

Attempts have been made to generalize that a transition from aquatic to aerial gas exchange is accompanied by a reduction in the Bohr effect but the recent work on transitional forms by Lenfant and Johansen does not support this idea (p. 55, 173,[138,139]). True *Neoceratodus* has a larger Bohr effect than *Lepidosiren* but that of *Protopterus* falls between ($\Delta \log p_{50}/\Delta pH = -0.62$, -0.24 and -0.47 respectively). In the amphibian series the trend is quite the other way—*Necturus* -0.13; *Amphiuma* -0.21; *R. catesbeiana* -0.29. It would seem safer to consider each case on its individual physiological merits.

Reversed Bohr effects

Finally, we may look briefly at those few cases where the Bohr effect is known to be reversed (positive) in the physiological range (p. 90). It has been suggested that these are examples of adventitious mal-adaptation. However, since the comparative study of respiratory pigments reveals so much advantageous adaptation and since the mechanism for modifying and selecting the desirable properties seems to work with such facility, one is tempted into the realms of pure speculation in order to find a teleological explanation.

A possible solution to the paradox, due to Redmond,[180] is illustrated by Fig. 9.15 based on some data for the marine gastropod *Busycon*.[85,176] If it be assumed that the unloading advantage is minimal, we can see a great potential advantage of a reverse Bohr effect for loading under conditions of periodic environmental oxygen deficiency which are associated with an increased ambient pCO_2. Steepening of the dissociation curve as a whole would favour the maintenance of a high arterial saturation in the face of falling external pO_2. Rising pCO_2 with falling pO_2 may often be encountered in aquatic environments where fermentation is pronounced. The surface crawling and superficial burrowing on mud-flats by *Busycon* and by the King-crab *Limulus* may expose them to just such conditions, though I am not aware of any attempt to establish this.

The case of the terrestrial gastropod *Helix pomatia* is less easy to account for. In this case rising pCO_2 and falling pO_2 are likely to be found in the pulmonary cavity which, in the interests of water conservation, is only opened at fairly long intervals. However, the reverse Bohr effect is only evident at pCO_2s above 10 mm (below this the effect is normal) and is then accompanied by a marked change in shape of the dissociation curve which becomes almost hyperbolic.[204] The result is that although at higher pCO_2s p_{50} decreases, p_{95} markedly increases. Pulmonary pCO_2 above about 10 mm would therefore inhibit loading, unless (as in the decapod crustacea) the respiratory cycle is confined to the lower half of the dissociation curve.

Redmond has put forward more recently[182,183] an alternative hypothesis on discovering reverse Bohr effects in two chitons (*Chiton tuberculatus* and *Acanthopleura granulata*) and two marine gastropods (*Fasciolaria tulipa* and *Fusitriton oregonensis*) which live on wave-swept rocks rather than on mud flats. He points

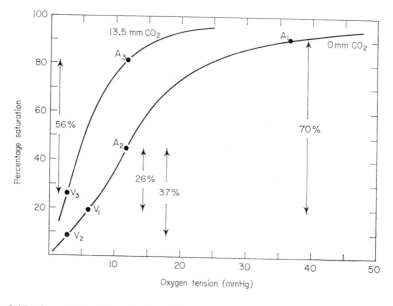

Fig. 9.15 Speculative interpretation of the reverse Bohr effect in *Busycon canaliculatum*. In well-aerated water arterial (A₁) and venous (V₁) tensions of 36 and 6 mm respectively ensure a turnover of 70% of oxygen capacity. If arterial pO_2 is reduced to 12 mm (A₂) in the absence of a Bohr effect turnover falls to 26% or to 37% if there is a drop of venous pO_2 to 3 mm (V₂). If fall in ambient pO_2 is accompanied by a rise in pCO_2 to (say) 13.5 mm, the whole curve is shifted to the left and 56% turn over can be achieved between 12 and 3 mm (A₃–V₃). (Dissociation curves from Redfield, Coolidge and Hurd[176]; data for points A₁ and V₁ from Henderson[85])

out that reverse Bohr effects have only been found in animals with open circulatory systems (p. 36) and that in such forms the movement of blood is partly a function of gross body movements and likely (especially when withdrawn into shells) to be somewhat erratic. In these conditions local increases in pCO_2 could occur in the more active tissues with resulting shift of the dissociation curve to the left in that region. This shift would encourage a diffusion of oxygen from less active regions of lower pCO_2. Thus the pigment could assume a role in facilitating diffusion at the tissue level. We shall return to the question of diffusion facilitation in the next chapter.

10 Oxygen Transfer and Storage Functions of Respiratory Pigments

Respiratory pigments are not confined to the straightforward type of transport functions described in the previous chapter. In addition to these we can recognize a number of uses in what can conveniently be called oxygen transfer systems and in a few cases a primary storage function.

THE MAMMALIAN PLACENTA

In the supply to the mammalian foetus, oxygen encounters an additional diffusion barrier in the form of a variable number of placental epithelia. For the foetus, maternal blood is the external medium and the placenta its respiratory organ. This poses a unique gas exchange problem involving the transfer of oxygen (and also of carbon dioxide) from one blood system to another. Two advantageous circumstances ensure that this transfer is effected with reasonable efficiency. In the first place there is in most species a crude kind of counter-current flow of the two bloods which encourages the exchange of gases in the same way as it does in the fish gill (p. 49). Even with this anatomical arrangement equilibration between the two bloods is often substantially incomplete; the pO_2 difference can be as much as 40 mm.

The second adaptation lies in the displacement of the foetal dissociation curve to the left with respect to that of the mother. The significance of this arrangement is well illustrated by some data for the sheep given in Fig. 10.1b. In this case the shift ensures that the foetal blood, leaving the placenta by the umbilical vein at a maximal pO_2 of about 40 mm less than maternal arterial blood, is able to achieve 90% saturation. The foetal venous blood, returning by the umbilical artery, is about 63% saturated. For an A-V difference in pO_2 of 20 mm in the foetal blood there has been a turn over of 27%. If there were no difference in the dissociation curves the same A-V difference (points a and v in the figure) would yield about 35%. In this particular example (at 80 days) the maternal/foetal shift seems to reduce the foetal oxygen turnover for the given drop in pO_2. However, as the pregnancy progresses, towards its full term at 150 days, the development of the placenta fails to keep pace with the increase in the oxygen needs of the foetus; the utilization of the maternal blood oxygen load increases, resulting in a lowering of the pO_2 both in the uterine vein and in the umbilical artery. In these conditions, the steeper slope of the lower part of the foetal curve pays off handsomely in superior pO_2 buffering.

The relatively large difference in oxygen affinity between maternal and foetal bloods in the sheep (difference in p_{50} about 25 mm) is presumably related to the magnitude of the diffusion barrier between the two bloods; the syndesmochorial type of placenta retains 5 of the 6 initial layers.[160] Barron and Meschia[12] estimated

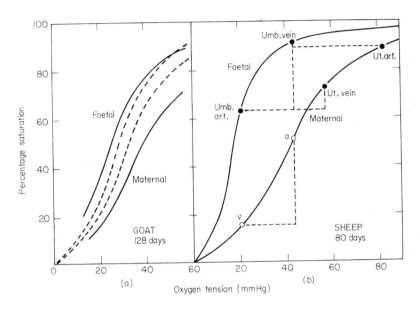

Fig. 10.1 The maternal/foetal shift. (a) In the goat a pregnancy acidosis moves the maternal curve to the right; the broken lines indicate the limits of the normal adult dissociation curve. (b) In the sheep the maternal blood shows a normal adult curve; the relationships of foetal and maternal arterial and venous bloods are shown at 80 days (full-term is c. 150 days); points a and v represent the conditions in foetal blood if the shift did not occur. (After Barcroft et al.[10] and Baron and Meschia[12] respectively)

the 'diffusion coefficient' of the placenta, which they defined as the number of ml of oxygen diffusing from maternal to foetal blood per min/kg of foetus/mm difference of pO_2 between the bloods. For the sheep at full term the value was 0.15, while for the rabbit it was 0.7. This substantially greater permeability of the rabbit placenta may be correlated with its haemoendothelial type (only the foetal endothelium surviving) and with a much smaller oxygen affinity difference (c. 5 mm difference in p_{50}).

In both these cases the maternal dissociation curve is similar to that of the non-pregnant female. This is not the case in the goat, where a large part of the maternal/foetal difference is due to a temporary shift of the maternal curve to the right (Fig. 10.1a); this results from a pregnancy acidosis—an unusual example of the functional significance of the Bohr effect. The shift is progressive and reaches a maximum later in term at about 128 days.[9] The goat also has a syndesmochorial placenta and the maximum foetal/maternal p_{50} difference is about 15–20 mm.

As a pointer to the dangers of making physiological deductions from studies on unphysiological materials, it may be mentioned that human foetal haemoglobin in solution gives a dissociation curve which lies to the right of that for a solution of the maternal pigment.[9]

GENERAL EMBRYONIC ADAPTATIONS IN VERTEBRATES

We have already noted that the foetal and adult haemoglobins in man are of distinctive types with substantial differences in amino acid sequences of the β-chains (p. 92). Some of these distinctions presumably form the structural basis for the difference in oxygen affinity (p_{50} difference is $c.$ 5 mm).[9] Although complete amino acid sequences are as yet known for few other species, simpler chemical techniques (notably electrophoresis) have revealed widespread differences between the haemoglobins of adults and embryos or larvae in many other vertebrates.[147] These 'intra-specific heterogeneities' are paralleled in the chick, a terrapin, the garter snake, the bullfrog, the spiny dogfish and lampreys, by oxygen affinity differences of the kind found in mammals. It seems likely, therefore, that the mammalian foetal/maternal shift represents a special exploitation of a more general situation—i.e. adaptation of vertebrate embryos to life in relatively adverse ambient pO_2 conditions, compared with their parents. While most of these blood heterogeneities probably rest on structural differences in the polypeptide chains, there is some evidence that in the garter snake (*Thamnophis*) the haemoglobins are identical but are provided with distinctive environments by the foetal and adult erythrocytes (Manwell[147], p. 225). Whatever their basis, the differences certainly reflect ontogenetic changes in haemopoiesis, with a sequence of no less than three haemoglobin types established in Man, goat, chick and bullfrog. There is probably also sequential use of distinct haemopoietic sites, e.g. in the frog, mesonephros, spleen and bone marrow.[63,153]

INVERTEBRATE OXYGEN TRANSFER SYSTEMS

It is not certain whether analogous oxygen transfer situations occur in invertebrates but there are a few possibilities where respiratory pigments occur in both vascular system and coelomic fluid. Manwell ([147,] p. 227) mentions that he found in the sipunculid *Dendrostomum* two such haemerythrins with different oxygen affinities but gives no details. A few polychaetes have haemoglobin in blood and in coelomic fluid—*Travisia*, *Terebella* and *Nephtys*—and a suggestive situation was found in the latter.[105] In *N. hombergii* both pigments are in solution (no coelomic corpuscles) and have virtually hyperbolic dissociation curves. At pH 7.0 the curves are indistinguishable but at pH 7.4 (the pH of freshly-drawn coelomic fluid) the vascular curve moves to the left, while the coelomic curve moves to the right with a reverse Bohr effect. Consequently, at the more alkaline (but probably physiological) pH the p_{50} values are 5.5 and 7.5 mm respectively (Fig. 10.3). This relatively large difference would be expected to facilitate transfer of oxygen from coelomic fluid to blood but it is difficult to see an adaptive significance. Detailed examination of the vascular system[30] shows that in *N. californiensis* there is a remarkable lack of capillaries, even in the massive dorsal and ventral longitudinal muscles. There are, however, very extensive systems of blind-ending diverticula on several of the main segmental blood vessels which are bathed by coelomic fluid. It is presumed that the coelomic fluid plays an important part in the distribution of oxygen but the flow would seem to be from the blood to the coelomic fluid rather than the other way if pigment transference is involved.

TRANSFER FROM BLOOD TO TISSUE

Storage role of myoglobin

A more ubiquitous kind of oxygen transfer system is that between vascular pigments and tissue pigments or myoglobins. Wherever the oxygen equilibria of such juxtaposed pigments have been investigated, it is found that the tissue pigment has the higher oxygen affinity. This seems to be as true for the haemocyanin/radular myoglobin relationship of chitons[145] as it is for the haemoglobin/myoglobin relationship of mammals (cf. Fig. 9.1, p. 98). As in the case of the maternal/foetal shift, the arrangement will encourage the transfer from vascular to tissue pigment at high percentage saturations even from capillary blood which has reached the venous level of pO_2. What is more difficult to establish in this case is the purpose of the intermediate binding system. The classical explanation, for the mammalian physiologist, ascribes to the myoglobin a transitory storage function. It is calculated that the typical myoglobin concentration of mammalian skeletal muscle holds a store equivalent to the oxygen need for not more than a second or so of vigorous activity. This could help to minimize anaerobic metabolism (a) during momentary local occlusion of capillaries by the intermittent contractions of groups of fibres and (b) during the short delay between the onset of vigorous contraction and the full opening-up of the capillary bed (p. 10). Both seem reasonable possibilities for vertebrate muscle fibres which make strong rhythmic or intermittent contractions and to such fibres myoglobin is restricted. But a third possibility has much to commend it, especially in relation to the diverse distribution of invertebrate tissue haemoglobins (p. 81).

Diffusion facilitation by myoglobin

This alternative idea of diffusion facilitation, stems initially from comparatively recent *in vitro* experiments of Wittenberg and of Scholander and Hemmingsen (see Hemmingsen[83] for a review of this topic). Atmospheric air, contained at various pressures in a high-pressure chamber, was permitted to diffuse through haemoglobin solution suspended in the pores of a Millepore filter, into a low-pressure chamber in which a moist vacuum was maintained. When the diffusion of the oxygen and nitrogen through the haemoglobin layer reached a steady state, the ratio of the two gases on the further (low) side of the membrane was determined. Since, besides the pressure gradient, the diffusion of each gas is proportional to its solubility and inversely proportional to the square root of its molecular weight (p. 4), an O_2/N_2 ratio of 0.49 would be expected if simple diffusion alone was occurring in each case. In the event, with air at atmospheric pressure on the 'high' side, the O_2/N_2 ratio on the low side was about 1. As the air pressure on the high side was lowered by stages to one-twelfth of an atmosphere the O_2/N_2 ratio rose to just over 4. When the membrane pores were filled with water or with plasma the ratio was about 0.56 at all pressures on the high side (Fig. 10.2). The movement of oxygen through the haemoglobin solution, therefore, rose from twice to eight times the rate which could be accounted for by simple

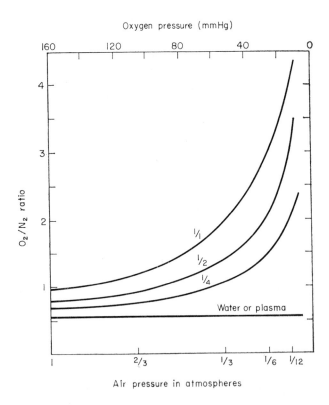

Fig. 10.2   Ratios of O_2/N_2 passing through a membrane with varying air pressures on one side and a vacuum on the other; membrane loaded with haemoglobin solution equivalent to whole blood, half or quarter dilution, plasma or water. (After Scholander[201])

diffusion. It was concluded that the actual oxygen flux consisted of two additive components (a) simple diffusion with rate dependent on pO_2 and (b) a 'specific oxygen transport' by the haemoglobin which is constant over a wide range of pO_2 gradients. The nitrogen flux (c), due to simple diffusion alone, is also pressure-dependent. If (a) and (c) are pressure-dependent and (b) is not, the ratio (a) + (b)/ (c) must steadily increase as total pressure on the high side is reduced, with pO_2/pN_2 remaining constant. In fact it was calculated that the specific oxygen transport (b) remained constant until the 'high' side pO_2 dropped below 20 mm.

The following additional points were established. With more dilute haemoglobin solutions in the membrane pores the specific oxygen transport was diminished roughly in proportion to the concentration. If the haemoglobin solution was solidified by the addition of 10% of gelatin, the specific oxygen transport was approximately halved while nitrogen diffusion was virtually unaffected. Filling the membrane pores with methaemoglobin (which does not bind oxygen) gave results identical with those for water or plasma. Using a somewhat different technique the effect was studied of varying the pO_2 on the 'low' side (formerly nil) of a haemoglobin-filled membrane. The specific oxygen transport proved to be maximal when the low side pO_2 was minimal. With a gradient of 20 mm from high to low sides, the specific transport was completely blocked when the 'low' side pO_2 rose to 10 mm. With a gradient of 80 mm, a low side pO_2 of 20 mm was needed for complete blocking of the transport. The p_{50} of the haemoglobin solution, measured in the membrane, was about 8 mm.[84]

In view of the evident need for the haemoglobin to bind the oxygen molecules, the apparent importance of the kinetic movement of the pigment molecules and of a degree of unsaturation of the pigment on the low side, Scholander postulated a 'bucket-brigade' or chain mechanism which enables the relatively static pigment to facilitate the diffusion of oxygen along a pO_2 gradient. A similar facilitation was also demonstrated with intact erythrocytes, with myoglobin solution (from the sea lion) and with haemoglobin solutions from the mackeral and a polychaete (*Thoracophelia*). A similar facilitation has also been found with haemerythrin solution from the sipunculid, *Golfingia*.[229]

On the basis of this and later work by a number of authors, strenuous efforts have been made to establish a quantitatively satisfactory model of the mechanism. These attempts have run into considerable difficulties as evidenced by the review of Kreuzer[120] who is forced to discount the 'bucket-brigade' hypothesis but emphasizes the importance of the diffusion of the oxygenated pigment. In considering the possible physiological significance of these *in vitro* observations Kreuzer discusses both the conflicting views on facilitated loading and unloading of oxygen by the red cell and the more likely diffusion facilitation role of myoglobin with or without an intermittent storage function.

Although the more difficult task of investigating diffusion facilitation *in vivo* with pigment-containing tissues has scarcely begun, it seems very probable that it will be found to occur; if it does the implications are obvious. Diffusion facilitation might be a supplementary function for vertebrate myoglobins but for invertebrate tissue haemoglobins it seems likely to be more important than the alternative classical role of oxygen store. In particular the idea makes more sense of the occurrence of haemoglobins in non-muscular tissues (p. 81). The pO_2 independence of the facilitation would be particularly useful in view of the very low tensions at which many invertebrate tissues must work.

STORAGE ROLE OF VASCULAR PIGMENTS

Having, perhaps, somewhat undermined the concept of oxygen storage by myoglobins we should consider whether a storage function is performed by any circulating pigments. The textbook accounts of invertebrate pigments abound with references to storage functions which have rarely been put to the test, experimentally.

Some estimates of storage capacity have been made; they are based on observed rates of oxygen uptake in relation to the product of oxygen capacity and blood volume. The resulting times are usually rather short compared with the period of likely exposure to oxygen lack. Several early writers ascribed a storage function to the haemoglobin of *Planorbis* but as we have seen above (p. 119), there is abundant evidence to show that the transport function is at least primary. Estimates of storage time for *Planorbis* range from 3 to 18 min.[21,136]

Arenicola and Nepthys

In the inter tidal sand-burrowing polychaete *Arenicola marina* the estimates range from 7 to 70 min. The upper value is promising but still short for an animal which may be prevented from irrigating its burrow for well over 6 hr. In any case, if the burrow becomes partly filled with air when the tide is out, the animal can probably resort to air-breathing.[222] There remains the possibility that the haemoglobin may serve as an oxygen store, during the pauses of up to 30 min, when irrigation is suspended in favour of other activities. An attempt to follow the changes in the pO_2 of burrow water during the phases of the activity cycle[223] would be useful. The situation might well resemble that already described for *Chironomus* (p. 114) where the pigment ensures the utilization of the burrow water during irrigation pauses and also serves as a short term store when the dissolved oxygen is exhausted. For *Arenicola* it has been estimated that the burrow water could hold as much oxygen as the blood itself.[107] The high affinity pigment (p_{50} is *c.* 2 mm[234]) is well-adapted to pick up most of this dissolved oxygen provided the gill diffusion barrier is not excessive. In this kind of situation (as with *Chironomus*) it would be difficult to disentangle transport and storage functions and not very meaningful to attempt it.

Another burrowing polychaete *Nephtys hombergii* has enough haemoglobin in the blood and coelomic fluid to provide the animal's oxygen needs for at most 15 min. This is a case where a realistic oxygen store would be very useful because, like *Arenicola*, *Nephtys* is often unable to irrigate its burrow for up to 6 hr or more when the tide ebbs. However, unlike that of *Arenicola*, the burrow is a very insubstantial affair; the opening to the surface collapses when exposed by the tide so that the animal is sealed up in the sand with access only to oxygen in the interstitial water. The pO_2 of this water at a depth of 10 cm or more on a clean beach does not exceed 7 mm. This is so low as to be virtually unusable however high the oxygen affinity of the pigment, since there is bound to be a gradient of at least 5–10 mm across the gills. *Nephtys* has in fact a pigment of relatively low oxygen affinity, having regard to the hyperbolic nature of the dissociation curve; it evidently does not even try to use oxygen at low tensions but must be exposed

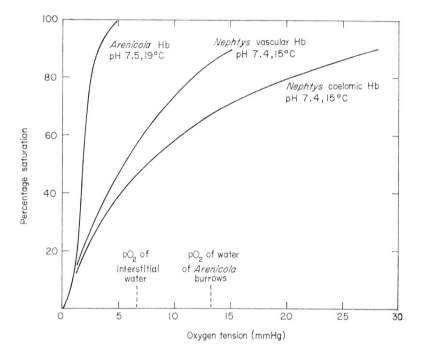

Fig. 10.3   Contrasting oxygen dissociation curves for two sand-burrowing polychaetes, *Arenicola marina* and *Nephtys hombergii*. Given a pO_2 gradient of about 10 mm across the gills, the high oxygen affinity pigment of *Arenicola* is probably capable of transporting oxygen from the residual water in the burrow (at 13.5 mm pO_2) but the pO_2 of interstitial water (6.7 mm) is too low to be capable of exploitation however steep the dissociation curve; this is the only oxygen available to *Nephtys* when the tide is out. (After Jones[105])

to regular periods of anaerobiosis. In the water of the *Arenicola* burrows on the same beach, pO_2 did not drop below about 14 mm even after 5 hr exposure. This tension is eminently usable given a high affinity pigment and a gradient at the gills not exceeding about 10 mm (Fig. 10.3). *Arenicola* may, therefore, be regarded as very well adapted (morphologically, physiologically and in behaviour) to its burrowing habit, while *Nephtys* is in all these respects very unspecialized.[105]

Storage v. transport

Consideration of these and other examples suggests that there is a limited sense in which any respiratory pigment will serve as an oxygen store, whenever ambient pO_2 falls low enough to prevent full saturation of arterial blood. The pigment, no longer binding its maximal amount of oxygen, may then be regarded as having given up part of its 'store' but this is quite incidental to its continuing role as a transporter. When ambient and arterial tensions fall so low that continued transport on a significant scale is impossible, the pigment will be virtually de-oxygenated and any residual storage function nil. It is therefore only sensible to speak of a circulating pigment having a primary storage function when the animal is suddenly cut off from external oxygen supplies with its store in a well-charged state.

ROLE OF COELOMIC PIGMENT

It can be argued that coelomic respiratory pigments should be regarded primarily as oxygen stores. Thus, in an extensive coelom, which assumes a respiratory function in the absence of a circulatory system, the fluid is well mixed by muscular contractions of the body wall and the pO_2 has a marked tendency to be uniform throughout. It is not possible, then, to distinguish the normal arterial and venous sides of the respiratory cycle with high and low tensions respectively. There will be local gradients into and out of the coelomic fluid at surfaces where oxygen enters or leaves the system but elsewhere conditions will be more or less uniform. So long as the uptake by the active tissues does not exceed the rate of intake from the respiratory surface this uniform pO_2 will also be steady. The presence of a pigment will be immaterial since in moving around the coelom its saturation will be virtually unchanged. However, if through increased oxygen demand or reduced ambient pO_2, uptake and intake get out of step, there will of necessity be a general drop in coelomic pO_2 and the pigment will come into operation as a store, tending to buffer the change.

To put the matter another way, the essential character of a transport pigment is to increase the oxygen capacity of the fluid which is being pumped from A to B (or rather to V) *and* to give up a superior volume of oxygen on arrival. So long as the mixing of the coelomic fluid is adequate to ensure that the uptake and intake gradients do not extend significantly into the body of the coelomic fluid, the pigment will only part with significant amounts of bound oxygen if the uptake rate exceeds the intake rate. Then it will be acting in the role of a store.

Urechis

This theoretical argument probably goes too far; it also lacks, at the moment, practical testing by the simple examination of oxygen uptake by normal and carbon monoxide treated specimens of suitable species. However, it is useful to review the existing data for the echiuroid, *Urechis caupo*, which may have a bearing on the case. The life of this worm, which occupies a U-shaped burrow in muddy sand between tide marks, has features in common with *Arenicola* and *Chironomus*. Hall[76] found that activity cycles include periods of rest, of moderate respiratory irrigation activity and of more energetic filter-feeding irrigation. The latter occurs in 10 to 20 min bursts making up about one-fifth of the total time. Oxygen uptake of worms in tubes is related to activity but not to the pO_2 of the water (down to 90 mm at least) but worms lying free in respiration flasks were pO_2 dependent below 120 mm; the importance of studying tubicolous animals in tubes is again apparent. Oxygen is principally take up via the thin-walled hind gut, which is filled by the muscular cloaca in a series of up to thirty inhalations followed by a single exhalation. Exhaled water contains a mean of 0.37 vols % of oxygen against 0.56 vols % for air-saturated water entering the burrow; hence the minimal hind gut pO_2 is about 100 mm.

Redfield and Florkin[177] took up the investigation of the pigment. The animal has no circulatory system but the coelom is packed with corpuscles containing haemoglobin. Coelomic fluid from well-aerated specimens has a pO_2 of not less than 75 mm and the pigment is fully saturated. The oxygen capacity is about 3.5 vols % and p_{50} about 12.5 mm at 19°C—a Bohr effect is lacking. With an average of 20 ml of coelomic fluid (about one-third of the weight of the worm) the oxygen requirement per minute amounts to only one-sixtieth of the total oxygen content of the coelom or about one-eighth of the dissolved oxygen content. The pigment is almost certainly functionless so long as *Urechis* pumps well-aerated sea-water through its burrow.

However, *Urechis* periodically rests from irrigation activity and remains totally inactive for 20 min to an hour or more. It is also prevented from irrigating when the tide goes out. During these periods its oxygen uptake will certainly be less than normal but the storage potential is of interest. Coelomic fluid oxygen would meet its active needs for at least 62 min; 54 min on combined, 8 min on dissolved oxygen. The storage function of the pigment would enable the animal to rest for nearly eight times as long as would otherwise be possible and this should comfortably carry it over the longest inactive periods, without even the necessity of ventilating the hind gut. Further, by virtue of the low oxygen affinity of the pigment, most of this oxygen store would become available before the coelomic pO_2 fell below 10 mm, a matter of some importance in the absence of a capillary circulation. When the tide is out, *Urechis* can also draw on some oxygen in the burrow water by periodic ventilation of the hind gut and this source is calculated to provide for about another 2 hr. As in the *Arenicola* burrow the minimum pO_2 of the stagnant water is about 14 mm after 4 hr but with an apparent gradient across the hind gut wall of about 25 mm under normal irrigation/ventilation conditions, the uptake from this low level will be rather restricted.

Sipunculus

Another group, where coelomic pigments compensate for the lack of a circulatory system, is the sipunculids. Unfortunately, very much less is known of the mode of life of these forms but some observations by Florkin[52] on the haemerythrin of *Sipunculus nudus* are of considerable interest. Gas exchange takes place across the general body surface and coelomic pO_2 for well-aerated specimens is only about 20 mm; the oxygen affinity is correspondingly lower than in *Urechis* ($p_{50} = 8$ mm at 19°C—no Bohr effect) and the pigment reaches 85% saturation. The coelomic fluid accounts for just over 50% of the total volume of the animal and its oxygen capacity is 1.6 vols % (total oxygen content 2.12 vols %). The animal is thought to make periodic excursions to a depth of 30 cm or more into the muddy sand. The chances of picking up oxygen through the unspecialized body wall and without irrigation while 'submerged' are virtually nil, but the coelomic fluid with its store of oxyhaemerythrin, fully charged at the surface, will increase the period of aerobic burrowing activity at least fourfold.

These observations on *Urechis* and *Sipunculus* do not of course provide a test of the storage-only hypothesis but they do suggest two cases which might repay re-examination from this point of view. The contrast in storage potential and oxygen affinity between the haemoglobins of *Urechis* and *Arenicola* certainly suggest a greater importance for the storage function in the former. It would, however, be a sterile academic exercise to attempt to draw a firm dividing line between storage and transport functions. The justification for discussing this matter at some length is the hope that this sort of attempt at critical and far-ranging comparative examination of particular cases may lead to a fuller understanding of the roles of respiratory pigments. At least it is to be hoped that enough has been said in this and the preceding chapter to refute the assertion by Wald ([213,] p. 369) that 'the hemoglobins that have arisen so sporadically among invertebrates of various orders are all storage hemoglobins'.

HAEMOGLOBIN OF PARASITES

The presence of haemoglobin in a number of endoparasitic forms, such as the pig roundworm *Ascaris lumbricoides* and the larva of the bot-fly *Gasterophilus intestinalis*, is well known but unfortunately not well understood. The very scattered literature in this field has been thoroughly reviewed and discussed by Lee and Smith.[134]

Positive identification of the pigment as haemoglobin has been made in about 20 species of nematodes with suggestions (based on colour) in as many more. Colouration also suggests that larvae of other species of *Gasterophilus* contain the pigment. In addition there are both positive and presumptive records among the digenetic trematodes but none among the cestodes. Respiratory pigments other than haemoglobin have never been found in parasitic forms.

Data on the physiologically important properties of these pigments are extremely limited, most work having been done on those of *Ascaris*. It does appear, nevertheless, that oxygen affinity is universally very high and where known $n = 1$. These facts taken together with the restriction to haemoglobin and the location in varied tissues (e.g. *Ascaris* body wall) suggest that the pigments have a myoglobin-like function with the emphasis on diffusion facilitation.

However, the perienteric fluid haemoglobin of *Ascaris* and of some other nematodes presents special problems. In *A. lumbricoides* the oxygen affinity ($p_{50} = c.$ 0.01 mm) is so high that it cannot be entirely deoxygenated by exposure to completely anaerobic conditions or to a vacuum. By contrast the body wall pigment has a p_{50} of about 0.5 mm. Lee and Smith have adduced evidence for the hypothesis that the perienteric fluid pigment serves as a metabolic store of haematin from which other haemoproteins can be synthesized and in particular is related to the needs of egg production. The concentration of the perienteric haemoglobin is markedly increased by the inclusion of porphyrin molecules in the medium, provided that they contain the vinyl group (Fig. 8.1) in the appropriate place.

Only in the larvae of *Gasterophilus*, which live in the stomach of the horse, is there a suggestion that the haemoglobin can permit a relatively aerobic existence by transporting oxygen at very low tension from air bubbles in the stomach contents. Even in this case p_{50} is said to be as low as 0.02 mm. The pigment is widely distributed in the tissues but is especially abundant in a peculiar organ made up of clusters of large cells arranged on tracheal branches and very well supplied with tracheoles.[128]

One other point seems well-established about all those parasite haemoglobins which have been sufficiently studied; contrary to earlier ideas, they are all endogenous to the parasites and structurally quite distinct from those of the hosts.

I I Respiratory Homeostasis and Regulation

As in other realms of physiological function, we may see the roles of respiratory mechanisms as contributing to a condition of homeostasis in which the concept of control by negative feedback is as valid as elsewhere.[90, 235] In a well-adapted animal the respiratory organs, the circulatory system and the blood should all combine to furnish the tissues with oxygen and eliminate carbon dioxide not only at the rate which is appropriate to the variation of internal demands from moment to moment but also, so far as possible, in the face of changing ambient conditions.

In earlier chapters we have noted in passing a number of features which contribute to this homeostasis but it is desirable to attempt a somewhat more systematic discussion of these regulatory mechanisms and to illustrate by a few examples the diversity of devices which have been developed in the various animal groups to this end.

EXTENT OF REGULATION

First we shall examine in a few cases the extent to which animals succeed in regulating their oxygen uptake. Systematic studies in this area are largely confined to the relationship between the overall oxygen consumption and ambient pO_2. We have already seen how decline in dissolved oxygen tension of the water is compensated, in the case of *Planorbis corneus* and *Lymnaea stagnalis*, by increased rate of uptake from the lung so that the total remains constant. With respect to declining dissolved oxygen, these snails are good 'regulators' so long as they have access to the atmosphere but if dependent on dissolved oxygen alone, uptake falls off steadily from 240 mm pO_2 downwards.[106] In nature, when access to the surface becomes difficult, *Lymnaea* responds by increasing the concentration of haemocyanin in the blood in order to exploit the pulmonary oxygen store to a greater extent.[110]

Most aquatic animals are not adapted to use atmospheric oxygen when dissolved oxygen tension declines. In this case it is frequently found that an optimal uptake can be maintained over some part of the upper ambient pO_2 range but a point is reached sooner or later where the regulatory mechanism proves inadequate and the uptake becomes markedly pressure-dependent. The oxygen tension at which regulation fails and the animal becomes a 'conformer' is called the critical tension (T_c). This concept is well illustrated by the goldfish, *Carassius*, as seen in Fig. 11.1. Oxygen uptake/oxygen tension curves have been determined at a variety of ambient temperatures and it is apparent that T_c rises with temperature.[64] On the same graph are included data for the toadfish *Opsanus* which is a conformer at all ambient pO_2s, at least up to 110 mm.[74]

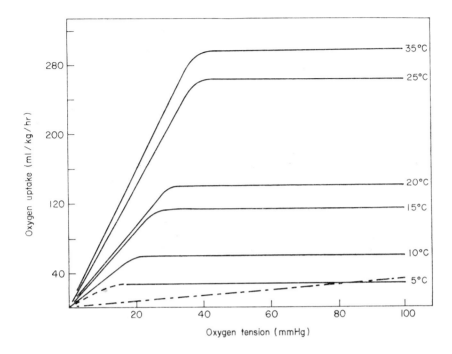

Fig. 11.1 The effect of temperature on the regulation of oxygen uptake in relation to changing ambient pO_2 in the goldfish. The uptake is held constant down to the critical tension, below which the animal is a conformer. T_c is progressively lower as the temperature falls. The lower broken line represents the complete conformity of the toadfish (uptake measured at 20°C), which is a very sluggish teleost capable of surviving 24 hr in oxygen-free water. (Goldfish curves from Fry and Hart;[64] toadfish curve from Hall[74])

It is unnecessary to review the great number of studies of this kind (see Prosser[174] for references) but it should be noted that conformity or lack of regulation is not simply a primitive character—the oxygen uptake of *Homarus vulgaris* is pressure-dependent right up to air-saturation.[210] Table 11.1 lists a number of regulators (with values of T_c) and conformers. The quoting of T_c values with some precision should not obscure the fact that a sharp change from regulation to conformity, as in the goldfish, is by no means the rule and the slope of the uptake/tension curve often increases very gradually.

A number of factors determine the value of T_c. The effect of temperatures on the regulatory powers of poikilotherms (illustrated by Fig. 11.1) is to be expected. As temperature-controlled basal metabolism rises, the lower limit of pO_2 for effective regulation is bound to rise also, unless the regulatory capacity is functionally unlimited. Similarly T_c is higher for active metabolism than for resting metabolism in the same species and in active species compared with sluggish species in the same group (see values for fishes in Table 11.1). Species adapted to life in swift flowing streams (e.g. nymphs of the mayfly, *Baetis*) show lesser powers of regulation than similar forms from ponds and lakes (e.g. *Leptophlebia* and *Cloëon*).[62] Berg has made extensive studies of oxygen uptake regulation in Danish freshwater snails (see [18] for references).

Within a single species short-term adaptation can also occur with consequent diminished dependence on pO_2 (e.g. *Chironomus plumosus*—see Fig. 9.8). Although some endoparasitic forms, such as *Trichinella* ($T_c = 8$ mm) have well

Table 11.1 Some examples of animals which regulate oxygen uptake with respect to ambient pO_2, with critical oxygen tensions (T_c) in mm Hg, ('regulators') and some which do not ('conformers'). (From data collected by Bishop[19] and by Prosser[174])

Regulators	T_c*	Conformers
Paramecium (ciliate)	50	*Spirostomum*
Tetrahymena (ciliate)	2.5	
Trypanosoma (flagellate)		
Pelmatohydra (hydrozoan)	60	Various sea anemones
Aurelia (scyphozoan)	120	*Cassiopea* (scyphozoan)
Tubifex (oligochaete)	25	*Nereis* (polychaete)
Lumbricus (oligochaete)	76	*Erpobdella* (leech)
Urechis (gephyrean)	70	*Sipunculus* (sipunculid)
Mytilus (lamellibranch)	75	
Helix (pulmonate)	75	*Limax* (pulmonate)
Loligo (squid)	45	
Cambarus (crayfish)	40	*Limulus* (king crab)
Uca (crab)	4	*Homarus* (lobster)
Cloeon (ephemerid nymph)	30	*Baetis* (ephemerid nymph)
Hyalophora (moth larva)	25	*Tanytarsus* (chironomid larva)
Tetraodon (puffer)	80	*Opsanus* (toadfish)
Stenotomus (the scup)	30	
Rana (frog)	45	*Triturus* (newt)

* The values of T_c must be accepted with caution since the transition from regulation to conformity is seldom sharply defined. Furthermore the shape of the oxygen uptake/tension curve is often influenced by degree of acclimation to abnormal pO_2s.

developed regulatory powers, facultative anaerobes generally seem to be conformers (*Fasciola, Schistosoma, Diphyllobothrium, Ascaris*), their capacity for anaerobiosis perhaps making regulatory powers unnecessary.[174]

Except for soil-dwelling animals, such as *Lumbricus* which is a poor regulator (see Fig. 9.3a), air-breathing animals are not normally subject to major variations in ambient pO_2, so the concept of critical tension is of little practical significance. They are, however, very much concerned with oxygen supply for varying levels of activity and well developed regulatory mechanisms are the rule. It might be asked why, if higher levels of oxygen uptake are possible, do not respiratory mechanisms work at top capacity all the time and thus save the trouble of regulation? The answer must be that high levels of uptake depend on high levels of ventilation or irrigation which are themselves, especially in aquatic animals, costly in energy terms. Furthermore, for air-breathing animals ventilation means water loss and this must be minimized in normal circumstances.

The site at which the pO_2 limitation becomes effective may be at the respiratory epithelium, in the oxygen transport system or in the metabolizing cell. The first two bottle-necks are well-known to offer scope for adaptation but for critical intracellular pO_2s also there is increasing evidence of adaptation (p. 159).

REGULATORY MECHANISMS

It is logical to divide the arrangements involved in compensatory adjustment of the oxygen supply lines into two classes. Those which are concerned with rapid adjustment to short-term (possibly minute by minute) changes in the supply and/or the demand, we shall refer to as regulation mechanisms and discuss below. Long-term adaptive or acclimative changes will be considered in later sections.

Regulation at tissue level

There is a degree to which increased use of oxygen by the tissue will of itself directly increase the rate of uptake from the medium by simply increasing the steepness of the oxygen diffusion gradient. In small animals which lack a circulatory system (p. 6) this is virtually the only 'mechanism' available; it is a simple matter involving only one gradient. In animals with a circulatory system two gradients are involved and with increased metabolism a greater arterial-venous pO_2 difference is created in the capillaries which, in turn, results in a steeper gradient and a greater uptake at the respiratory epithelium. The scope of this two-stage adjustment is greatly enhanced by the pO_2-buffering action of respiratory pigments (p. 98).

Somewhat less direct than this but equally 'automatic' is the osmotically controlled movement of fluid in the tracheolar endings of insects, which has already been discussed (p. 74) and its analogue in the opening-up of the tissue capillary beds as the result of accumulating anaerobic metabolites in other animals.

Regulation in mammals and birds

In most animals with circulatory systems (and in the tracheal system of insects) these simple direct controls are supplemented by further mechanisms which act remotely from the sites of oxygen utilization and commonly come under some measure of nervous control. Broadly, we are concerned here with control of (a) rate of circulation in the vascular system and (b) rate of ventilation or irrigation of the respiratory surfaces by the external medium. Separately or together, variation in these parameters may also incidentally but significantly alter the oxygen utilization from the medium.

The rhythmic functions of hearts and respiratory muscles are basically, in vertebrates and cephalopods at least, under reflex nervous control and it is upon the basic rhythms that the excitatory (or inhibitory) effects of variable respiratory factors are imposed. As is well-known, the mammalian breathing rhythm involves stretch and relaxation proprioceptors in the lungs which alternately cause central nervous (medulla) inhibition and excitation of the inspiratory muscles.[32] Respiratory contractions of the mantle in cephalopods are under analogous reflex nervous control.[51]

Our concern is mainly with the factors which modify the basic patterns rather than with the generation of the patterns themselves. In almost all air-breathing animals the primary respiratory stimulant is carbon dioxide which can accumulate to excite appropriate receptors if ventilation and/or circulation are inadequate. Thus the chemosensitive areas of the mammalian brain are situated bi-laterally in the ventro-lateral regions of the medulla (distinct from the median medullary respiratory centre) and are thought normally to react to locally increased hydrogen ion concentration caused by excess pCO_2. Both the rate and amplitude of ventilation are increased by stimulation of these centres. In addition both the chemosensitive centres of the medulla and the peripheral chemoreceptors (carotid and aortic bodies) are sensitive to change in the arterial pH per se. The hyperventilation caused by the latter stimulus is only found in abnormal conditions of acidosis and perhaps in very severe exercise. The carotid and aortic bodies also function as pO_2 receptors but significantly increased ventilation from this cause is only found when the oxygen concentration of inspired air falls below 10%.[32,157] This is a matter of normal physiological significance only at high altitude.

While the regulatory significance of variations in pCO_2, pH and pO_2 is well-understood for the resting subject, the cause of hyperventilation (hyperpnoea) in exercise is still a mystery. Ventilation rate (amplitude times frequency) in well-trained athletes may rise to 15–20 times the resting level yet arterial and alveolar pCO_2 and blood acidity remain constant or in heavy work show a slight decrease; arterial pO_2 remains even more constant but may eventually show a slight rise. (Work to exhaustion may cause a slight fall in pO_2, increase in pCO_2 and fall in pH). What is more, local tissue level changes in these parameters also fail to induce hyperpnoea.[32] Some recent work suggests that the primary stimulus to exercise hyperpnoea may be neural[113] and that the impulses originate in the working muscles rather than in the brain.[161]

Not unnaturally, regulation of respiratory movements is less well-known in other vertebrates. The inspiratory/expiratory rhythm of birds is based on reflexes similar to those of mammals but with the addition of an air-movement receptor in the trachea which appears to reinforce the inhibition of inspiration until expiration is complete. Control of ventilation in birds also appears to follow the mammalian pattern but there is evidence of an additional chemo-receptor in the lungs themselves which responds to change in lung pCO_2. In connection with temperature regulation there is also an additional 'panting' centre in the medulla.[193]

Regulation in aquatic vertebrates

In aquatic animals carbon dioxide is a less appropriate respiratory stimulus since its ready elimination makes it an unreliable indicator of the oxygen supply position. Accordingly, there is a marked tendency for oxygen concentration to take over the role of primary respiratory stimulant. This is very evident in the amphibia where pO_2-dependent hyperventilation is at least partly mediated by the carotid gland. However, in species adapted for prolonged submergence (*R. esculenta* and *R. temporaria*) reflex hyperventilation in response to low arterial pO_2 can be suppressed and the oxygen content of the lungs can be reduced to zero. Fall in alveolar pO_2 also induces opening-up of the pulmonary capillary bed. Appropriately, variation of ambient pO_2 and pCO_2 also regulates the number of capillaries open in the cutaneous circulation.[63]

In *Neoceratodus* and *Lepidosiren* reduced pO_2 in the water acts as a stimulant to increased irrigation of gills and/or ventilation of lungs respectively. This response is only found in juvenile *Protopterus* which are more dependent on their gills and capable of prolonged survival without access to air; the adults alone among fishes seem quite insensitive to dissolved pO_2 but are stimulated to increased ventilation by bodily exposure to air or by breathing oxygen deficient gas mixtures. Elevated pCO_2 in the water causes depressed branchial irrigation and increased pulmonary ventilation in mature *Protopterus*.[139]

Knowledge of teleost respiratory regulation is scanty. Again practical control is probably primarily a result of decreased oxygen tensions though sensitivity to pCO_2 changes can be demonstrated and shows some apparently adaptive variations. Thus the air-breathing electric eel has a high sensitivity to pCO_2[131] and fishes from swamp waters (where ambient pCO_2 is usually high) are markedly less sensitive to carbon dioxide than those from well-aerated waters.[89] Fishes seem to have additional pO_2-sensitive receptors in the gill epithelia and in elasmobranchs these show an inhibitory influence which is removed by section of the ninth and tenth cranial nerves.[174] A similar operation produces a lessened response to lowered pO_2 in the tench.[89]

Regulation of utilization

The possibility of increasing oxygen utilization from the respiratory medium does not normally arise in mammals because the whole control mechanism is orientated to the rigid stabilization of alveolar pO_2 and pCO_2. Expired air therefore bears the same relationship to inspired air under all but the most severe conditions of respiratory stress. A slight increase in utilization probably occurs at high altitudes because the anoxemia (reduced oxygen content of arterial blood) increases alveolar ventilation with the object of bringing about a closer identity between alveolar and inspired air (p. 157, 159).

Branchial respiration would seem to offer more possibilities for increasing utilization. Van Dam[36] examined this question very carefully in the eel and in a trout and found that in well-aerated water a utilization of up to 80% occurred. At lower pO_2s this value remained unchanged down to about 40 mm; below this level, utilization tended to fall. Fish, like lung-breathers, therefore depend on increased irrigation and circulation to keep up oxygen intake in the face of falling ambient pO_2 as well as in sustaining high levels of activity. On reflection, this is logical because by adjusting irrigation rate to achieve maximal utilization at all levels of activity and ambient pO_2, the animal does not have to expend more energy than is currently necessary in the work of the respiratory muscles.

Some aquatic animals with fairly high minimal utilization do increase the level with fall in ambient pO_2. Table 11.2 gives some data to illustrate the point for

Table 11.2 The effect of decreasing ambient oxygen concentration on the irrigation rate, utilization and oxygen uptake rate in the lobster, *Homarus vulgaris*, at a temperature of 15°C. (Data selected from Thomas[210])

Oxygen concentration (ml/l)	Irrigation rate (l/hr)	Utilization (%)	Oxygen uptake (ml/g/hr)
5.78	9.77	31.0	0.045
4.63	9.22	36.6	0.041
3.23	9.52	47.9	0.038
2.44	9.56	55.1	0.033

Homarus vulgaris.[210] In this case irrigation does not increase and the utilization improvement presumably rests on increased branchial circulation; the regulation cannot prevent a gradual fall in oxygen consumption, however. *Homarus* is in fact a conformer. On the other hand, increased oxygen uptake with temperature depends on both increased irrigation and increased utilization (Table 11.3). A

Table 11.3 The effect of increasing temperature on irrigation rate, utilization and oxygen uptake rate in the lobster, *Homarus vulgaris*, at an ambient oxygen concentration of 5.3 ml/l. Although oxygen concentration is constant, pO_2 increases with temperature. (Data selected from Thomas[210])

Temperature (°C)	pO_2 (mmHg)	Irrigation rate (l/hr)	Utilization (%)	Oxygen uptake (ml/g/hr)
8.0	129	6.0	34.5	0.032
13.5	144	8.4	40.0	0.051
17.5	154	9.8	41.0	0.060
20.5	163	11.7	43.0	0.076

similar situation is found in *Octopus* where decline in ambient oxygen concentration to 25% of air-saturation results in a utilization improvement from 35 to 70%; in this case irrigation rate also increases fourfold and uptake is maintained.[228]

Aerial and aquatic regulation in invertebrates

Like amphibia and fish, aquatic invertebrates show a general picture of greater respiratory sensitivity to oxygen lack than to carbon dioxide excess. Increased irrigation at low ambient pO_2 in *Octopus* was noted above but increased ambient pCO_2 (of doubtful natural significance) also causes increases in both frequency and amplitude of respiratory movements. This animal seems to be more sensitive to carbon dioxide than most aquatic animals.[174]

The basic difference between terrestrial and aquatic animals as regards the respiratory sensitivity to changes in pO_2, is well illustrated by comparison of similar animals from different habitats. In isopods and amphipods, acceleration of movements of the pleopods when the pO_2 of the medium was below 50% air-saturation was greatest in brackish-water species. *Gammarus locusta* and *Idotea basteri*; less in marine and freshwater species, *Cymodoce emarginata* and *Melita palmata*; *G. pulex* and *Asellus aquaticus*; and nil in semiterrestrial species, *Orchestia gammarellus* and *Ligia italica*. This sequence was thought to correspond to increasing stability of ambient pO_2.[216] In the terrestrial pulmonates *Limax*, *Arion* and *Helix* the opening of the pneumostome is stimulated by carbon dioxide and at 3 to 5% it remains permanently open.[174] This is in marked contrast to the air-breathing but aquatic snails *Planorbis corneus* and *Lymnaea stagnalis*, where carbon dioxide does not accumulate in the lung during the dive and so cannot act as a respiratory stimulus to bring the animals to the surface (p. 119). There is reason to believe that in this case the respiratory stimulus is a combination of reduced pulmonary pO_2 *per se* and loss of buoyancy of the shell complex.[106]

Regulation in insects

Respiratory regulation in insects is complex. Reference has already been made to the osmotic withdrawal of tracheolar fluid (p. 74) but there are also mechanisms for regulating spiracular opening and tracheal and air sac ventilation. Predictably, carbon dioxide is the primary stimulant for terrestrial forms.

Spiracular opening may be controlled by direct action of carbon dioxide on the closer muscle or there may be additional nervous control of the direct response to the gas. In fleas there is evidence that opening is a direct result of falling pO_2, while the duration of the open phase is determined by rate of drop in pCO_2. Spiracular fluttering in the Cecropia pupa (p. 73) is caused by hypoxia acting centrally and mediated by the spiracular nerves, while full opening of the spiracles periodically is a direct effect of high pCO_2 ($> 6\%$). It seems likely that where neural effects are found, local sensitivity to carbon dioxide can be modified by the frequency of motor impulses from the appropriate ganglion and that the latter, in turn, can be influenced by a variety of factors including dessication and temperature as well as by hypoxia or carbon dioxide accumulation.[156]

Ventilation movements are essentially rhythmic and there may be pacemakers situated in abdominal ganglia. There is also evidence for co-ordination by sensory inputs from inspiration and expiration proprioceptors. The activity of the ventilation centres can be modified by a negative feedback of raised pCO_2 or with less sensitivity by lowered pO_2. In some forms at least (*Blaberus*), the stimulant effect of carbon dioxide is not specific but is paralleled by any weak acid.[156]

RESPIRATORY ACCLIMATION

The regulatory mechanisms described above can cope with transient changes in oxygen demand or supply but an important further aspect of respiratory homeostasis is found in the ability of many individual animals to make longer term adaptations to environmental respiratory stress. Some of these are briefly discussed in this and the following sections.

Hypertrophy of respiratory organs

Perhaps logically, the first line of defence against persistently lowered ambient pO_2 would be development of the area of the respiratory epithelium. Some cases in which this does occur have already been mentioned. In frogs and salamanders and also in the male lungfish *Lepidosiren* (p. 55) hypertrophy of existing or new gill structures has been described. In the bug *Rhodnius*, both tracheae and tracheoles develop and become more densely distributed to the more important organs and tissues if ambient pO_2 is lowered (p. 74), though to what extent this contingency may occur naturally, is doubtful. Somewhat analogous changes also occur in the lungs and tissues of mammals at high altitude (see a later section).

Response of respiratory pigments

The second line of defence lies in the circulatory system and especially in the oxygen-carrying properties of the blood. It is well known that prolonged exposure to relatively low ambient pO_2 stimulates the synthesis of haemoglobin in a number of animals but not in others. Fox reported[60] significant increases in the haemolymph concentration of haemoglobin in a number of phyllopod crustacea, including *Artemia* and four species of *Daphnia*, and in two species of chironomid larvae. Outside the arthropods, positive responses were obtained from freshly hatched but not from adult *Planorbis corneus*. Three annelids, *Arenicola*, *Scoloplos* and *Tubifex* did not respond. In a number of cases the effect was shown to be reversible.

In *Artemia* haemoglobin synthesis was also shown to be stimulated by high external salinities and studies have been made of its contribution to oxygen uptake and survival in oxygen deficient waters.[69] Fox and his co-workers also made a notable series of studies on the functional role of the pigment in *Daphnia* mainly by measurement of performance of such functions as filter-feeding in relation to varying pigment concentrations and ambient pO_2s (see Fox[60] for references). This work has been summarized elsewhere.[107] Increase in the haemoglobin content of the blood and in the myoglobin content of muscle in mammals at high altitudes is referred to later (p. 156, 159).

In only one species so far has an increase in haemocyanin concentration been found to result from exposure to respiratory stress. This is the rather special case of *Lymnaea stagnalis*, where access to the water surface for refilling the lung may be more difficult in some habitats than in others (p. 122).

Because the oxygen affinity of many respiratory pigments is closely adapted to providing optimal saturation at prevailing arterial pO_2 (p. 100), variation in oxygen affinity is of potential acclimative significance. However, since the basic affinity of specific pigments is genetically determined, the possible acclimation of individuals might depend on varying some aspects of the pigment's vascular environment which is capable of modifying the functional oxygen affinity. This possibility has, in a sense, been exploited in those female mammals where the difference in maternal and foetal oxygen affinities is in part due to a Bohr effect shift to the right of the maternal oxygen dissociation curve (p. 133 but see also p. 134). This represents an acclimation of the mother for the benefit of the foetus. Prolonged shifts of plasma pH might be detrimental on other grounds but there is perhaps a theoretical possibility of differentially raising the pH of the erythrocyte; red cell pH is normally about 0.3 units lower than that of the plasma.[20]

An alternative possibility for individual acclimation is suggested by the observation of very wide oxygen affinity variations among some of the abnormal human haemoglobins. Values of p_{50} (at pH 7.4 and 37°C) range from 12 mm in haemoglobin Yakima to 70 mm in haemoglobin Kansas. Associated with this variation there seems to be a general inverse correlation between oxygen affinity and oxygen capacity with the result that in the resting state at least, the arterio-venous percentage difference in oxygen content and the mixed venous oxygen tension tend to be stabilized about the normal levels (4 to 5 vols % and 35 to 45 mm). Oxygen capacity is thought to be regulated through the influence of renal venous pO_2 on erythropoietin production.[163] If, as is known to be the case in some mammals and also in decapod crustacea, the blood contains a variety of molecular species, the increased production of one or more of these pigments with the suppression of others and an appropriate adjustment of oxygen capacity could form a powerful mode of acclimation to variation in arterial pO_2.

Tolerance of low oxygen tensions

Many studies of acclimation to low ambient pO_2 indicate an increased tolerance, often with maintained oxygen uptake. Some of these responses appear to involve an increased capacity for removing oxygen from the medium by methods which are as yet undisclosed. This is the case, for example, in the speckled trout, *Salvelinus fontinalis*, where the 95% tolerance level for low oxygen concentration is 1.9 mg/l in normal animals, while for acclimated individuals the lowest tolerance limit is 1.05 mg/l.[202]

ANAEROBIOSIS

The ultimate recourse in acclimation (or in failure to regulate) to an oxygen deficient environment is the development of a greater tolerance of anaerobiosis. Tolerance is largely a genetically determined factor but there are a number of cases where acclimation has been demonstrated and doubtless there are many more in which it does occur. Since animal tissues lack pyruvate decarboxylase, anaerobic glycolysis cannot yield ethanol, so significant amounts of carbon dioxide cannot arise directly from metabolism without oxygen.* Respiratory gas exchange is virtually in abeyance and anaerobiosis, therefore, strictly falls outside the scope of the present work. However, as short periods of anaerobiosis may have subsequent gas exchange consequences and as partial or short-term anaerobiosis is probably a commonplace, especially among less highly organized invertebrates, a short summary of the essentials may not be out of place.

Strict anaerobiosis is rare, being confined to a few groups of bacteria and possibly the intestinal flagellates of termites etc. These obligate anaerobes are not only incapable of utilizing oxygen but are actually poisoned by oxygen at quite low partial pressures. Some animals are facultative anaerobes, capable of using oxygen when available but otherwise tolerant of complete anoxia or extremely low ambient pO_2 for very long periods. Here one can include metazoan parasites, most intestinal protozoa (such as rumen ciliates) and a variety of forms adapted to largely anoxic non-parasitic environments, such as tubificid worms.

The great majority of animals are strict aerobes, incapable of living for protracted periods in the complete absence of oxygen. This group we may divide into two categories: (a) those which are able to tolerate complete oxygen lack for some hours, but not indefinitely, such as frogs, some reptiles and many invertebrates; and (b) those which are highly intolerant of complete oxygen lack but are capable of a certain amount of anaerobic metabolism in selected tissues such as muscle (see p. 32). The latter category includes birds and mammals, many adult insects and cephalopods. None of these categories is sharply delimited and a continuous spectrum of tolerance would give a more accurate picture.

The factors which determine tolerance, measured as survival time with complete or partial or selective anaerobiosis, are diverse. Sluggish animals tend to be more tolerant than related active forms and hibernators are more tolerant than non-hibernating individuals of the same species. In highly tolerant animals, especially the facultative anaerobes, there is usually a complete excretion of the acidic metabolites e.g. lactic, valeric, caproic, butyric and propionic acids, which are the universal end-products (in animals) of anaerobic carbohydrate metabolism. Such a procedure represents a complete wastage of a very large proportion

* A number of reactions of non-carbohydrate substrates are known to yield carbon dioxide anaerobically[6,22] but they are of marginal importance from an energy-releasing standpoint.

of the energy potentially derivable from the substrate under aerobic conditions of complete oxidation. This is presumably a matter of little consequence to gut parasites.

Oxygen debt

Less tolerant forms, particularly those in the last category of strict aerobes, retain more or less of the acidic end-products and when oxygen becomes available again, use the energy from complete oxidation of part of the stock-pile to re-synthesize the remainder into a more suitable storage form, usually glycogen. This resynthesis demands oxygen in excess of normal aerobic requirements, hence the concept of 'oxygen-debt'—an exalted post-anaerobic consumption.

Oxygen debts, like tolerance itself, are extremely variable and all degrees of repayment are found. Measured oxygen debt may not be proportional to the amount of acid retained, if slow complete oxidation for current energy provision predominates over resynthesis. Since there are also varying degrees of excretion and retention, neither the repaid debt nor the retained acid necessarily reflects the total anaerobic metabolism. Facultative anaerobes, of necessity, effect a complete excretion of acidic metabolites; indeed it may be their specialized capacity for excretion which gives their superior tolerance.

Some of the better adapted forms in our first category of strict aerobes also excrete completely, or almost completely, e.g. *Nereis, Urechis, Chironomus plumosus* and *C. thummi* (but not *C. bathophilus*). Others in this category repay extensive oxygen debts at varying rates (e.g. *Mya, Planorbis, Tenebrio, Planaria, Lumbricus*, cockroaches and grasshoppers) as do the least tolerant forms in the last category. In non-excretors anaerobic survival is finally limited by the concentration tolerance of the end-products. In mammals at least the limit of short-burst high activity (e.g. performance in middle distance running) is determined largely by muscular fatigue due to lactic acid accumulation. In man the limit of oxygen debt is of the order of 10 l, which may require an hour or more for its complete repayment.

Abnormal respiratory quotients

During partial (or complete) anaerobiosis excessively high (or infinite) RQs may be found as a result of the buffering of accumulating acid, either through the release of normally bound carbon dioxide, e.g. tissue and body fluid bicarbonate, or by reaction with calcareous skeletons such as the valves of lamellibranchs. Post-anaerobic RQs are often lower than normal because carbon dioxide is being re-bound in order to restore the sources depleted by acid buffering—increased alkali reserve. For a more extensive but succinct summary of the significance, especially of 'abnormal' RQs the reader may consult the account by Bishop.[19]*

* No attempt has been made to document fully this very general account. The interested reader should consult the accounts by Bishop[19] and Prosser[174] for summaries and references and von Brand[22,23] for notable reviews of anaerobiosis in invertebrates.

F

ADAPTATION AND ACCLIMATION TO HIGH ALTITUDE*

The most extreme adjustments to hypoxic stress in mammals are found at high altitudes and have long been a matter of interest to respiratory physiologists. We have not yet arrived at a full understanding of the solutions to this problem but many interesting facts are established. Some distinction must be made between the regulation shown by visitors to high altitudes in which a complete state of acclimation is reached in the course of some weeks or months and long-term adaptation, achieved by native residents over many years.

Adaptation of respiratory and circulatory mechanisms

The basic problem arises from the fall in total atmospheric pressure, which is halved for every rise of 5500 m (18000 ft), and the proportionate fall in ambient pO_2. A number of studies have been made of indigenous populations at high altitude in the Andes at settlements up to 5000 m and one recent study by Hurtado,[95] in which a comparison was made with residents at sea-level, will be summarized. Measurements were made on natives of the mining town of Morococha at 4540 m and residents of Lima at sea-level.

The key to the adaptation is illustrated in Fig. 11.2, which shows the striking differences between populations in respect of the total gradient of pO_2 between tracheal air (i.e. atmospheric air saturated with water vapour) and mixed venous blood (representing the lowest pO_2 outside the tissues). The tracheal pO_2 at this altitude is less than the total gradient at sea-level and this fact dramatically highlights the need for adaptive mechanisms. The most striking economies are achieved (a) across the alveolar epithelium (1.5 v 9 mm) and (b) between the arterial and venous sides of the circulation (10.5 v 45 mm). These values are for resting subjects where BMR was the same in the two groups.

The values of the principal respiratory parameters which provide an explanation of this striking difference, are presented in simplified form in Table 11.4. Increased respiratory frequency is responsible for the hyperventilation and the volume of air ventilated per litre of oxygen consumed is up by about one-third. Sensitivity of the chemoreceptors seems to be adjusted in order that the system continues to regulate in the normal manner but at lowered alveolar and arterial pCO_2s (p. 148). The total lung volume is only slightly larger but there is a substantially increased residual volume, so that the alveoli are substantially larger at expiration. This, together with a permanent dilation of the capillary bed (known from animal studies) would encourage exchange across the alveolar epithelium.

The oxygen capacity of the blood is improved by a 64% increase in the red cell count, which permits the arterial-venous cycle to operate over a reduced percent-

* No attempt is made in this section to distinguish systematically between natural and experimental acclimation, both relatively short-term effects, but the changes due to very long term exposure to hypoxia are distinguished by the term 'adaptation'.

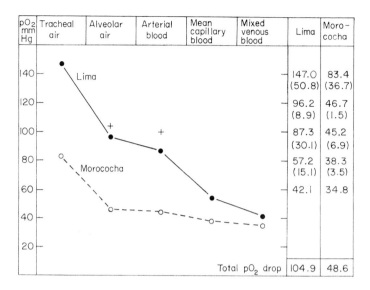

pO_2 mm Hg	Tracheal air	Alveolar air	Arterial blood	Mean capillary blood	Mixed venous blood	Lima	Morococha
140						147.0 (50.8)	83.4 (36.7)
120						96.2 (8.9)	46.7 (1.5)
100						87.3 (30.1)	45.2 (6.9)
80						57.2 (15.1)	38.3 (3.5)
60						42.1	34.8
40							
20							
Total pO_2 drop						104.9	48.6

Fig. 11.2   Comparison of the resting metabolism components of the pO_2 gradient from tracheal air to mixed venous blood in the residents of Lima (sea-level) and the natives of the town of Morococha (alt. 4540 m) In the right-hand columns are the actual pO_2 values and the differences (in brackets). The alveolar epithelium gradient for the sea-level subjects is rather greater than the mean usually given; standard values of pO_2 for alveolar air and arterial blood are shown by +. (After Hurtado[95])

age saturation range and hence at much lower pO_2s, on a steeper part of the dissociation curve. It is interesting also to see that the high altitude dissociation curve is slightly to the right of the sea-level curve (p_{50} of 26.9 v 24.7 mm) at a common pH of 7.40. However, these values are slightly suspect because the standard value of p_{50} at pH 7.4 for man is 27.0 mm. A decrease in oxygen affinity would also be in contrast to the findings of significantly increased affinity at high altitude in the llama and the vicuna.[75] Hurtado also found in his altitude subjects a smaller difference between calculated mean capillary and observed mixed venous blood pO_2s. This could be accounted for by an increase in the tissue capillary bed, which has been found experimentally in guinea pigs.

When a comparison was made between the two groups at work the high altitude subjects showed a considerable superiority. Each group, in its own milieu, was asked to run to exhaustion on a treadmill at a constant speed of 132 m per min (c. 5 mph) up a gradient of 11%. The mean tolerance time for the sea-level subjects was 34 min ($\equiv$4.6 km), for the altitude subjects 59 min ($\equiv$7.9 km). Over their greater total time, the latter were characterized by greater pulmonary ventilation (now including greater tidal volume); lower oxygen consumption per kg-m of work; lower pulse rate and smaller rise in blood pressure; lower oxygen debt and lower lactic acid accumulation. In virtually every way more physical work

Table 11.4 Principal respiratory parameters for residents of Lima (sea-level) and natives of the town of Morococha (alt. 4540 m), at rest and in exhaustive exercise. (After Hurtado[95])

Resting

	Lima	Morococha
Ventilation (l/min/m²)	4.8	6.4
Respiratory rate (/min)	14.7	17.3
Total lung capacity (l)	6.5	6.96
Tidal volume (l)	0.60	0.59
Vital capacity (l)	5.00	4.88
Residual volume (l)	1.50	2.07
Ventilatory quotient (l vent/l O_2 consumed)	32.7	42.5
Red cell volume (ml/kg)	37.2	61.1
Haemoglobin (g/kg)	12.6	20.7
p_{50} (mm Hg) at pH 7.40	24.7	26.9
Arterial % saturation (pO_2)	98 (87)	81 (45)
Venous % saturation (pO_2)	80 (42)	65 (35)
Arterial pCO_2 (mm Hg)	40	33
Arterial plasma pH	7.41	7.39
Oxygen capacity(mM/l)	9.30	12.29

Exercise to exhaustion

	Lima	Morococha
Duration (min)	34.2	59.4
Ventilation (l/min/m²)	37.5	42.2
O_2 consumption (l/min/m²)	1.33	1.17
O_2 consumption (ml/kg-m)	2.66	2.43
CO_2 production (l/min/m²)	1.27	1.11
Calories (/min/m²)	6.70	5.81
Respiratory rate (/min)	37.2	36.4
Tidal volume (l)	1.77	1.83
Pulse rate (/min)	183	160
Blood pressure—resting	116/79	93/63
Blood pressure—exercise	138/71	97/65
Oxygen debt (l)	2.96	2.39
Lactic acid (mEq/l)	1.35–6.37	1.30–3.19
Net efficiency %	19.9	22.2

was performed with less departure from their own standards of resting metabolism by the high altitude natives than by the residents at sea-level (Table 11.4). The greater efficiency of the work performance (mechanical calories/total calories − basal calories) and the failure of the respiratory adaptations entirely to prevent a fall in mixed venous pO_2 make it likely that the high altitude subjects also enjoy some adaptations at the cellular level.

A comprehensive review of work on mammalian adaptations to high altitude has been given by Stickney and van Liere.[206]

Adaptation and acclimation at tissue level

Barbashova[8] has drawn attention to a very large number of anomalous findings on the parallelism between degree of acclimation to hypoxia and the extent of change in the conventional respiratory parameters. She concludes, like Hurtado, that there must be, both in acclimation and in adaptation, additional tissue level adjustments and she finds in the literature much evidence to support a number of potentially important features. Among these are the ability of isolated tissues of acclimated animals to utilize oxygen down to lower limits of pO_2 and of acclimated whole animals to maintain higher oxygen consumptions at lower ambient pO_2. This is explained by a number of observations of increases in activity of certain cell components such as cytochrome oxidase, FAD, various dehydrogenases and, in homoiotherms, temporarily in tissue carbonic anhydrase. One of the most widely reported changes is an increase in the concentration of myoglobin in both heart and skeletal muscle; this occurs both in short-term acclimation and in animals reared at high altitudes. The oxygen storage role is usually stressed but in this context the increase would seem to lend strong support to the diffusion facilitation hypothesis (p. 135).

Barbashova[8] has also stressed the widespread evidence for increased anaerobic glycolysis in acclimated organisms and their isolated tissues, with, in some cases, reduced oxygen consumption. This is seen a ssupplementary rather than as an alternative to utilization of oxygen at low tissue tensions. Increases in phosphocreatine and ATP activity in skeletal muscle and of ATPase in skeletal muscle, heart, liver and kidney have also been found in hypoxic acclimation. For many of these cellular changes as well as the respiratory system adjustments, the biochemistry and physiology of muscular training provide significant parallels.

Acclimation of respiratory mechanisms

Short-term acclimation of respiratory gas exchange differs somewhat from full adaptation to altitude hypoxia. The principle immediate responses are those of increased ventilation (both respiratory frequency and tidal volume) which reaches a maximum after a matter of days or weeks according to altitude. This is accompanied by substantial falls in arterial pCO_2 and a more alkaline plasma. During this period an adjustment in the sensitivity of the carbon dioxide chemoreceptors occurs to enable the regulation to be controlled by lower level variation in pCO_2 rather than by pO_2 as in the first few days.[115] As haemopoesis (and perhaps also myoglobin increase) proceeds, the extreme ventilatory responses diminish and blood pH and acid-base levels tend partly back towards normal sea-level values.

Knowledge of hypoxic acclimation and adaptation outside the mammals is extremely fragmentary. In the S. American ostrich and the Bolivian goose the oxygen capacity of the blood is higher than in sea-level birds, while in this goose oxygen capacity is also increased.[75]

ADAPTATIONS TO DIVING

No review of comparative respiratory physiology would be complete without some account of the adaptations which enable many air-breathing vertebrates to survive prolonged periods underwater. Many secondarily aquatic reptiles, birds and mammals exhibit striking phylogenetic adaptations of normal patterns of ventilation, gas exchange, circulation and metabolism which enable them to feed below the surface. Table 11.5 includes, amongst other things, estimates of the maximum dive duration in a small selection of diving birds and mammals with data from the pigeon and man for comparison. The outstanding contributions in this field are linked with the names of Irving and Scholander.* As a result of their work and that of others, the general principles are clearly established; they may be summarized under three heads:

(i) Oxygen storage factors and respiratory properties of the blood.
(ii) Oxygen economy factors including cardiovascular and respiratory responses.
(iii) Metabolic adjustments.

Oxygen storage and blood properties

Increased relative lung volumes do not generally contribute to greater oxygen stores (Table 11.5), probably because, in order to avoid the dangers of caisson disease (due to liberation, on rapid surfacing, of excess nitrogen dissolved under pressure in the blood), most divers exhale before submerging. Whales, which submerge without exhalation, have unusually small lungs in relation to their size and it is calculated that under the hydrostatic pressure at 100 m depth the whole of the gas is compressed into the volume of the lung dead space where no exchange will occur. Some recent lung volume determinations in pinnipeds by Lenfant et al.[141] are unusually high even for divers, more than twice that for man. The extent of exploitation of these larger volumes is unknown.

Blood volumes, relative to body weight, are in most cases higher than in non-divers but the excess is very variable. The oxygen capacity is also raised in a number of cases, especially among some pinnipeds (seals and sea elephants) but not notably among the whales. In the latter group the main increase in oxygen storage capacity appears to lie in very high concentrations of myoglobin in the

* There is no attempt at complete documentation of this section; reference should be made to the classic review of Scholander[199] and to the more recent reviews of Andersen,[4] Lenfant[137] and Elsner.[44]

skeletal muscles, a factor which shows a significant increase in all diving mammals where measurements are available. Oxygen stores are therefore greater in most divers than in non-divers but the increases are generally not dramatic and the emphasis falls on different factors in different groups (Table 11.5).

In a few cases attempts have been made to estimate the duration of dive which could be sustained aerobically by these oxygen stores assuming a resting metabolic rate. These estimates compare unfavourably with known maximum dive durations (Table 11.5) so it is clear that the actual dives, which in most cases will be active periods, cannot be accounted for on this basis.

Some other blood parameters show variations from values found in terrestrial animals. The oxygen affinity is sometimes lower, notably in the larger whales (except the sperm whale) and in most of the pinnipeds, a circumstance which may facilitate the transfer of oxygen to the tissues. Probably more significant, especially in rapid repayment of the oxygen debt (see below), is the greater Bohr effect which is found in all but the larger whales. The elevated values of $\Delta \log p_{50}/\Delta$ pH lie in the range -0.53 to -0.80 compared with -0.50 for man and -0.37 for the elephant. These high values are the more remarkable if the normal size dependence of the Bohr effect is borne in mind (p. 126). Abnormally large Bohr effects have also been found in the crocodile and the alligator. The carbon dioxide dissociation curves of diving mammals are normal but there is generally among divers a superior buffering capacity (see below). Even when not diving a greater part of the blood oxygen load is turned over than is normal in mammals, as evidenced by the vols % utilization figures in Table 11.5.

Oxygen economy and cardiovascular adjustments

In all diving species of mammals, birds and reptiles immersion results in a very pronounced bradycardia, which takes the form of a prolonged diastolic phase and is due to vagal inhibition. Bert, in the earliest significant study of diving physiology (1870), found a drop from 100 to 14 beats per min in the duck. In the seal, *Phoca vitulina*, the rate drops from 110 to 9 beats per min (Fig. 11.3). The extent of cardiac retardation varies from species to species and according to whether the submersion is forced or spontaneous. Less pronounced immersion bradycardia has also been found in a number of terrestrial forms (including snakes, sloths, armadillo, dog, pig and man) and in fishes removed from water. Since stroke volume normally remains constant, cardiac output decreases in proportion to heart rate. Mean arterial blood pressure, however, is often maintained at a normal level and this points to a widespread peripheral vasoconstriction. Where a pressure fall does occur it is more pronounced during diastole than in systole, so pulse pressure is maintained or even increased.

There is now abundant direct evidence of drastically reduced peripheral blood flow in a number of mammals and birds. Ischemic tissues include most of the skeletal muscles and skin, the gastro-intestinal system (except for the oesophagus in ducks), the kidneys and many glands (but not liver, thyroid and adrenals). On the other hand, coronary and cerebral circulation is unimpaired or even increased.

Table 11.5 Values for a number of respiratory parameters in a selection of diving birds and mammals compared with the pigeon and man. Calculated dive duration refers to the period for which the estimated oxygen stores would support resting metabolism aerobically. Oxygen utilization is here given as the % O_2-content difference between inspired and expired air. Carbon dioxide combining capacity is the concentration of total CO_2 in whole blood when pCO_2 is 40 mm. Buffer capacity is the change in HCO_3^- concentration to shift pH one unit. Values marked * from Lenfant et al.[141] (see comment on lung values in text); other values collected by Andersen,[4] Scholander,[199] Lenfant,[137] Elsner[44] and Sturkie.[207]

	Max. dive duration (min) Obsd.	Calc.	Lung vol. (ml/kg)	Tidal vol. (ml/kg) (as % of total)	% O_2 utilization	Blood vol. (% B.W.)	O_2 capacity (vols %)	O_2 affinity (p_{50} at pH 7.4)	Bohr effect (Δ log p_{50} ΔpH)	CO_2 combining capacity (mM/l)	Buffer capacity (mM/l/ pH)	Myoglobin (g%)
Duck *Anas platyrhyncos*	15	4		(15)	5–7	10.0	16.9	50				
Penguin *Pygoscelis papua*	7	3				9.0	20.7					
Guillemot *Uria troile*	12					12.3 –13.7	26.0					
Puffin *Mormon fratercula*	4					11.3 –12.0	24.0					
Pigeon *Columba livia*	1			(10)	6.5	7.0	21.2	35				
Porpoise *P. phocoena*												
P. communis			69	54(73)	7.5–9.5	15.0	20.8	24.5	–0.60	18.2		
Bottlenosed dolphin *Tursiops truncatus*			66	59(89)	8–10	7.1	18.0 –21.9	26.8	–0.66	21.1	43.2	
Killer whale *Orcinus orca*							21.5 –22.6	30.7	–0.74	20.1	42.8	
Sperm whale *Physeter catodon*	75						18.5 –29.1	26.5	–0.48			

F 2

Species													
Fin whale *Balaenoptera plupalis*	30	17	29	25(86)	8–10								
Bottlenose whale *Hyperoodon rostratus*	120	36	25	22(88)	8–10	14.1							
Harbour seal *Phoca vitulina**			91				13.2 –15.9	26.4 –29.3	31.0	–0.53	19.1	40.2	5.5
Hooded seal *Cystophora cristata*	18	6					12.0	26.6	29.5		20.1		7.7
Sea lion *Eumetopias jubata**			110				9.2	17.5 –20.1	32.0	–0.80	18.4	32.0	2.4
Sea elephant *Mirounga angustirostris*							12.0	28.0 –39.0	30.5	–0.63	20.0	41.8	
Walrus *Odobenus rosmarus**			116				10.6	23.4	34.2	–0.53		34.0	3.0
Manatee *Trichechus manaus*	15		51	29(57)	7–10			17.2					
Man *Homo sapiens*	2.5		50	8(16)	4–5		6.2 –7.0	20.6	27.0	–0.50	21.5	24.0	0.8

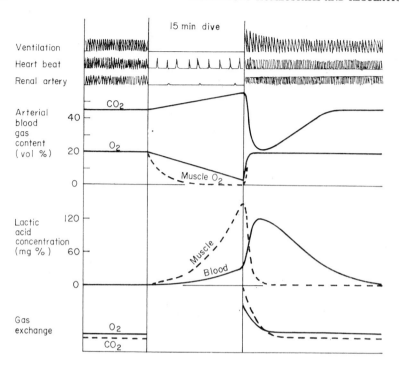

Fig. 11.3 Schematic representation of some of the cardiovascular and respiratory changes which occur during and after a dive of about 15 min duration in a seal. The rates of ventilation, heart beat and renal artery pulse are not to scale; an approximate indication is given for the levels of arterial blood gas and lactic acid concentration. (Freely adapted from Scholander[199])

The immediacy of vasoconstriction responses leaves little doubt of the neural nature of the regulation; hormones or accummulated metabolites are not involved, at least at the onset. Similar indications have also been found in non-diving mammals including man; in these cases immersion of the nasal region, as well as breath holding, is a necessary stimulus to maximal systemic responses. Notwithstanding the thoroughness of these vasoconstriction arrangements to ensure priority for the brain and heart, there is some evidence that the brain of the Weddell seal is somewhat less sensitive to oxygen lack than is normal in mammals.[45]

Ventilation rate in divers is not completely insensitive to arterial carbon dioxide as is often stated. Seals and ducks have both been shown to increase the respiratory minute volume with physiological increases in pCO_2 but they differ from terrestrial forms in the extent of the response. Breathing 7.5% carbon dioxide causes approximately a sevenfold increase in ventilation in man but in the duck it is only doubled. The suspension of respiratory movements during the dive depends on an immersion reflex mediated by receptors in the nasal region; this reflex is not weakened by increasing arterial pCO_2, as is voluntary breath holding.

Several unique morphological features of diving mammals are related to the cardiovascular adaptations described above. In addition to a number of unusual venous sinuses in the abdomen and a much enlarged posterior region of the inferior vena cava, there is commonly a well-developed striated muscle sphincter in the vena cava at the level of the diaphragm. There is good evidence from the elephant seal that these arrangements provide a venous store of well-oxygenated blood in the abdomen which can be admitted to the thoracic circulation as required. Also found in all diving mammals are extensive circulatory plexuses and *rete* systems. Those associated with flippers, fins and tail flukes are usually regarded as counter-current exchangers involved in heat conservation but others are probably arterio-venous shunts. The thoracic plexus of whales seems to be specifically involved in supply to the brain via an unusual arterial network overlying the dura mater.

Metabolic adjustments

Since calculated oxygen reserves are insufficient to support observed durations of dive aerobically and since arterial oxygen content decreases in a linear manner with time and dive duration seems to be limited by final arterial oxygen content, two metabolic situations are possible. The selective distribution of available oxygen to tissues which are sensitive to hypoxia either leaves the remainder to a predominantly anaerobic metabolism or there is sharp reduction in the metabolism of these underpriviledged tissues. There is evidence that both these possibilities are involved.

It has been observed in seals that the oxygen store of skeletal muscle is depleted much more rapidly than that in arterial blood and reaches a virtual zero level long before termination of the dive. The high myoglobin content of the muscles of many divers can retard this depletion locally but because of the ischemia cannot contribute to the needs of other regions. Also of the highest significance is the very much greater rate of accumulation of lactic acid in the muscle than in the surviving circulation. On emmersion the muscle lactic acid level falls sharply and there is a massive rise in the blood concentration of this metabolite. The blood level declines slowly as the oxygen debt is paid off (Fig. 11.3). The pattern of blood lactic acid changes is less pronounced in the alligator and the guillemot, suggesting a less effective restriction of the peripheral circulation.

Rapid repayment of the oxygen debt constitutes an essential part of successful adaptation and several factors contribute. The very superior tidal volume which may exceed 80% of total lung volume, compared with less than 20% in man, is undoubtedly very important. The large tidal volume makes possible an abnormally high utilization of alveolar oxygen (Table 11.5). In addition high oxygen capacities and superior Bohr effects help in the transport of the excess oxygen needed at this time. Equally important is the restriction of disturbance of the acid-base balance by the flooding of the blood with acidic metabolites. Here we find one of the most consistent adaptations, at least in mammals, since the buffering capacity is always much higher than in man (Table 11.5). The finding of unusually high plasma protein levels in the killer whale and the failure of buffering capacity to correlate with haemoglobin concentration suggest that an unusual pattern of buffering may be involved (cf. Fig. 12.1, p. 170).

In addition to a marked reliance on anaerobic metabolism by non-sensitive tissues, there is some evidence that total energy metabolism is depressed during quiet dives. Thus in seals, manatee, duck and alligator the excess oxygen uptake after prolonged but quiet dives is much less than would be expected on the basis of pre-diving oxygen consumption. In ducks there is a marked drop in body temperature when the head only is immersed in water, in spite of an improvement in insulation by peripheral vasoconstriction; a fall in body temperature during quiet total immersion has also been found in a seal. Such depression of metabolism presumably represents a suspension of non-essential functions and would be masked by the anaerobic heat production of skeletal muscles during active dives.

Andersen has drawn attention to the fact that 'the physiological adjustments seen in diving are not defensive mechanisms unique among vertebrate divers. Their adaptation to environment lies rather in the perfection of a fundamental facility common to all vertebrates.'[4] This concept applies as well to the cardio-vascular adjustments for oxygen economy and their consequences as to the inadequate attempts to provide superior oxygen stores. The only apparently unique features are the minor morphological variations which assist in the exploitation of the cardiovascular adjustments.

12 Transport and Elimination of Carbon Dioxide

The problems involved in the elimination of respiratory carbon dioxide are, in a sense, less severe than those which arise in ensuring adequate oxygen uptake. Because of the thirty times greater solubility and 1.4 times higher molecular weight of carbon dioxide, diffusion co-efficients for this gas are about twenty-five times higher than for oxygen (p. 5). This means that for a net flux equal to that of oxygen (if RQ $= 1$) diffusion gradients of pCO_2 twenty-five times less than those of pO_2 should suffice. In the absence of anaerobic fermentations, short-fall of oxygen deliveries to animal tissues will of necessity diminish carbon dioxide production proportionately, though other acidic metabolites may be produced (p. 154). Arrangements which permit the uptake of a given amount of oxygen at the respiratory surface and its distribution via the tissue capillaries will be more than adequate to ensure the diffusion and transport of the corresponding carbon dioxide in the opposite direction.

CARBON DIOXIDE BUFFERING

For reasons which are illustrated by the data of Table 12.1, interest in carbon dioxide elimination centres mainly on the means of transporting substantial quantities of this acidic substance without undue change in blood pH. If carbon dioxide were transported only in solution in the blood, a turn over of 10 vols % would involve a venous-arterial pCO_2 difference of about 160 mm at 37°C (cf. dissolved carbon dioxide curve in Fig. 12.2). This would entail a pCO_2 in excess of 160 mm in the tissues and an excessive V-A pH change in the blood, whereas in fact, large quantities of carbon dioxide are actually transported at low pCO_2 and with little change in pH, thanks to the presence of relatively complex pCO_2 and pH buffering systems.

The nature of the carbon dioxide system in the blood has been succinctly summarized by Wolvekamp[233] whose review may be consulted for detailed references. The following reactions are possible:

$$CO_2 + H_2O \rightleftharpoons H_2CO_3 \rightleftharpoons H^+ + HCO_3^-$$

and

$$CO_2 + OH^- \rightleftharpoons HCO_3^- \rightleftharpoons H^+ + CO_3^{--}$$

The second sequence occurs to an appreciable extent only at reactions above pH 8.5 (at pH 9 about 5% of absorbed carbon dioxide as in the form of carbonate)

Table 12.1   Carbon dioxide transport in a selection of invertebrates and vertebrates. Total carbon dioxide content of blood in vols %; pCO_2 in mm Hg; buffer value expressed as ΔCO_2 vols%/ΔpH in the cycle. Data from various authors as indicated; those for man are not standard values but the results of a study on a single subject at rest and at work with oxygen uptake at 7 times the resting level. For comparison a hypothetical pCO_2 differential is given for a 10 vols% turnover by a blood consisting of normal saline.

		Saline	Busycon[85]	Panulirus[180]	Loligo[176, 178]	Raia[39]	Duck[219]	Man at rest[20]	Man[20] at work
CO_2 content	venous	10	14.3	10.62	8.27	10.84	55	52.0	—
	arterial	0	12.8	10.0	3.98	7.70	47	48.2	—
	V-A	10	1.5	0.62	4.29	3.14	8	3.8	—
pCO_2	venous	158	3.3	5.6	6.0	2.6	65	45.4	54.8
	arterial	0	2.0	5.0	2.2	1.3	54	40.0	38.0
	V-A	158	1.3	0.6	3.8	1.3	11	5.4	16.8
pH	venous		7.79	—	—	7.67	7.20	7.40	7.35
	arterial		7.96	—	—	7.82	7.23	7.43	7.28
	A-V		0.17	0.04	0.13	0.15	0.03	0.03	0.07
Buffer value			8.8	15.15	33.0	20.9	266	127	—

and only about 0.1% of absorbed carbon dioxide is in the form of carbonic acid. Accordingly, we are concerned principally with dissolved carbon dioxide, bicarbonate ions and concommitant hydrogen ions.

The system may be treated quantitatively by use of the Mass Action Law and a practically useful derivation is the Henderson-Hasselbalch equation: $pH = pK + \log[HCO_3^-] - \log[CO_2]$ where pK is the reciprocal exponent of the carbonic acid dissociation constant K (cf. pH). The maximal buffering capacity of the bicarbonate system is found when $[HCO_3^-]$ equals $[CO_2]$, that is when $pH = pK$. But the value of pK in mammalian bloods is about 6.1, whereas pH is about 7.5. It is clear that the simple carbonic acid/bicarbonate system is inadequate as a buffer. The system is also inadequate to account for the large amounts of carbon dioxide which are known to be transported.[233]

The functional arrangements in fact depend additionally on the presence of other weak acids. Although blood phosphates play a minor part, much more important are the blood proteins. Having many free ionizable basic ($-NH_2$) and acidic ($-COOH$) groups, these molecules are amphoteric but since blood pH is normally well on the alkaline side of the isoelectric point, the molecules may be represented as proteinic acids —H.Pr. Thus:

$$H.Pr + NaHCO_3 \rightleftharpoons Na.Pr + H_2O + CO_2$$

In addition a proportion of the absorbed carbon dioxide is transported in direct combination with free amino-groups on the blood proteins, forming carbamino-compounds or carbamates, which can also dissociate:

$$Pr.NH_2 + CO_2 \rightleftharpoons Pr.NHCOOH \rightleftharpoons Pr.NHCOO^- + H^+$$

Clearly the pK of the Henderson-Hasselbalch equation is no longer a function of the simple dissociation constant of carbonic acid and if the equation is to be used as a means of calculating pH from determinations of $[HCO_3^-]$ and $[CO_2]$ a composite value of pK^1 should be determined for the blood in question. In fact, pH values are now very often obtained directly, by careful use of the hydrogen electrode.

CARBON DIOXIDE TRANSPORT IN VERTEBRATE BLOODS

From the elements discussed above the overall situation in vertebrate bloods may be represented in the form of a diagram as in Fig. 12.1. Diffusing in solution across the capillary wall into the plasma, carbon dioxide reacts slowly with water to form carbonic acid which rapidly dissociates. A limited amount of carbamate is formed, which also dissociates. The liberated hydrogen ions are buffered to a slight extent by phosphates but mainly by association with the negatively charged carboxylic groups of the plasma proteins.

Much the larger part of the loaded carbon dioxide diffuses into the erythrocytes because within the cells an enzyme, carbonic anhydrase, catalyses the formation of carbonic acid and so favours the production of bicarbonate. Free hydrogen ions in this case are buffered by the haemoglobin. The build-up of bicarbonate within the cell, which would tend to slow up the reaction of carbon dioxide with water and hence impede its entry into the cell, is minimized by the diffusion of this ion out into the plasma. Consequent upon the impermeability of the erythrocyte membrane to cations the distribution of diffusible anions is governed by a Donnan equilibrium:

$$[HCO_3^-]_c \times [Cl^-]_p = [HCO_3^-]_p + [Cl^-]_c$$

Increase of $[HCO_3^-]_c$ tends to disturb the equilibrium, which is maintained by outward migration of this ion and inward migration of chloride—the so-called 'chloride shift' or Hamburger phenomenon.

Substantial amounts of carbamate are formed within the cells by reaction with haemoglobin and once again the liberated hydrogen ions are buffered by the haemoglobin.

The Haldane effect

In the buffering of all these hydrogen ions by haemoglobin an important reciprocal relationship is involved. As we saw earlier (p. 91) the normal Bohr effect reflects the reduced oxygen affinity of respiratory pigments at lower pH due to the pigment protein then carrying a smaller net negative charge (weaker acid). The converse of this situation is that as haemoglobin unloads its oxygen in the tissue capillaries, the total negative charge on the protein increases and the acceptance

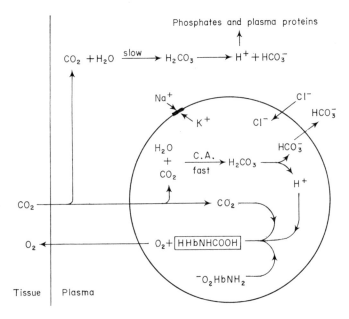

Fig. 12.1 Schematic representation of the inter-relation of oxygen and carbon transport in vertebrate blood. Reactions shown occur in the tissue capillaries; in the gills or lungs the arrows are reversed. Focusing of deoxygenation, carboxylation and hydrogen binding on deoxycarbaminohaemoglobin emphasizes the interdependence of these processes. However, more haemoglobin molecules are involved in oxygen transport than in hydrogen buffering and carbamate formation (even when R.Q.=1) because (a) a proportion of carbon dioxide molecules do not enter the erythrocyte and (b) 27% of carbon dioxide taken up forms carbamate, which is only slightly dissociated to form hydrogen ion. Hydrogen ions and oxygen molecules are bound at different sites on the molecule. (For further explanation see text)

of hydrogen ions is facilitated. Since unbuffered hydrogen ions in addition to lowering pH will also hinder the reaction of carbon dioxide, the equilibrium carbon dioxide content of deoxygenated blood is greater than that of oxygenated blood at any given pCO_2. This phenomenon is known as the Haldane effect and is manifest in the comparison of the carbon dioxide dissociation curves for oxygenated and deoxygenated human blood in Fig. 12.2.

There is a general correlation between magnitude and direction of the Bohr and Haldane effects in any particular blood but it is often not exact. The dis-

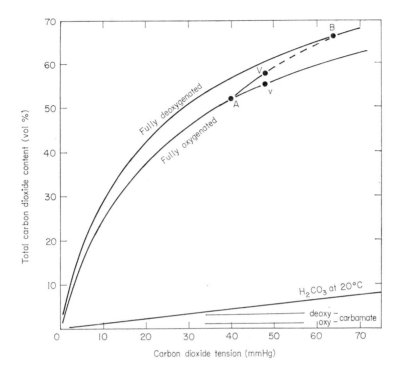

Fig. 12.2 Carbon dioxide dissociation curves for fully oxygenated and deoxygenated human blood to illustrate the significance of the Haldane effect which increases the resting turnover of carbon dioxide by the amount V–v. During exercise point V moves nearer to B. Below the dissolved oxygen line is an approximate representation of carbamate content in oxygenated and deoxygenated blood; carbamate concentration depends almost entirely on the degree of oxygenation of the haemoglobin. (Jones[107])

crepancies may, in some cases, reflect the fact that the Haldane effect has an alternative component, the inhibitory effect of oxygenation upon carbamate formation. This direct combination of carbon dioxide with blood proteins is very little dependent on pCO_2 in the physiological range but is very much dependent on percentage deoxygenation (Fig. 12.2). As a consequence of the two aspects of the Haldane effect, the turnover of carbon dioxide in the blood of man for V-A pCO_2 difference 48–40 mm is approximately doubled.

Distribution of carbon dioxide in the blood of man

Table 12.2 illustrates the way in which the various aspects of carbon dioxide transport and buffering are represented in the blood of man. It is apparent from this table and from Fig. 12.2, that arterial blood still contains a large amount of carbon dioxide. This reflects the high alveolar pCO_2 and the failure of the blood to come to equilibrium with the true external medium; the full load is given up when blood samples are equilibrated with zero pCO_2 but this is not true of some

Table 12.2 Distribution of carbon dioxide in the blood of man. A comparison of the states of plasma and cells in venous and arterial blood with respect to dissolved CO_2, carbamate and bicarbonate and to the net negative charge on the proteins. All values are in mMoles/l of whole blood in the resting subject. (After Comroe[32])

	Venous blood		Arterial blood		V-A difference	
Whole blood						
Total CO_2	**23.21**		**21.53**		**1.68**	
Plasma						
Total CO_2	16.99		15.94		1.05	
dissolved CO_2		0.80		0.71		0.09
bicarbonate ion		16.19		15.23		0.96
Protein −ve charge	7.80		7.89		−0.09	
Red blood cells						
Total CO_2	6.22		5.59		0.63	
dissolved CO_2		0.39		0.34		0.05
bicarbonate ion		4.41		4.28		0.13
carbamate		1.42		0.97		0.45
Protein −ve charge	21.15		22.60		−1.45	

other vertebrate bloods (see below). The pattern of transport in man is clear from the venous-arterial differences in Table 12.2.

Although in absolute terms the amount of venous blood carbamate is only about 6% of the total load, this fraction is (by virtue of the Haldane effect) much the most labile and in turnover contributes about 27% of the whole, while changes in dissolved carbon dioxide (8%) and bicarbonate (65%) account for the remainder. In consequence of the chloride shift most of the bicarbonate is transported in the plasma—equivalent to 57% of the total carbon dioxide turn-over. That most of the buffering of hydrogen ions occurs in the erythrocytes can be seen from the greater V-A drop in net negative charge on the red cell proteins as compared with plasma proteins.

Although the bloods of all animals may be presumed to have buffering powers adequate to their activities, even at rest but more particularly during exercise some change of pH does occur; indeed, some aspects of respiratory regulation depend on such changes (p. 148). In a comparison of subjects at rest and at work (on a stationary bicycle with oxygen consumption seven times the resting value) the plasma V-A pH difference rose from −0.026 at rest to −0.073 at work. The corresponding differences in the red cells were −0.008 and −0.035.[20] The venous figures were obtained from mixed venous blood and so are likely, in the working subjects, to underestimate the rise as it actually occurs in the capillaries of the working muscles. It is interesting to note that the red cells are somewhat better buffered than the plasma in both cases and that the burden of the bigger change of pH during work falls more heavily on the plasma.

This system provides an outstanding example of the finely adjusted interdependence of physiological mechanisms. Increase in haemoglobin concentration not only permits a higher rate of aerobic metabolism by increasing the oxygen transport capacity of the blood but at the same time provides the means of transporting and buffering the corresponding increase in carbon dioxide. Furthermore, the natures of the reciprocal oxygen and carbon dioxide-binding mechanisms are such as to provide mutual enhancement with more rapid exchange and equilibration in the tissues and in the lungs. A more detailed account of carbon dioxide transport with extensive references may be found in the review by Roughton.[246]

Carbon dioxide transport in other vertebrates

Although there are some differences in detail, there is no reason to believe that carbon dioxide transport and buffering mechanisms of other vertebrates differ in essentials from those described above. The true external medium is, with few exceptions, a carbon dioxide sink in which the pCO_2 is always low and virtually unaffected by the respiration of organisms. Together with the high diffusion coefficients of carbon dioxide, this sink ensures an adequate flux of the gas with very modest internal V-A pCO_2 differences so long as the carbon dioxide capacity of the blood is adequate.

However, actual internal pCO_2s are dependent on the nature of the respiratory organs. As we have seen, in lung-breathers the elevated alveolar pCO_2 results in the labile fraction of carbon dioxide being superimposed on a substantial non-labile fraction.* In the duck, venous and arterial pCO_2s are 65 and 54 mm respectively. In gill-breathers, on the other hand, branchial blood comes very close to equilibrium with the true external medium and the non-labile pCO_2 is generally low. Thus venous and arterial pCO_2s are 2.6 and 1.3 mm respectively in the skate *Raja ocellata*.[39] In active fishes venous pCO_2 may rise to 10 mm.[175] However, in some freshwater vertebrates not all the blood carbon dioxide comes off when pCO_2 is reduced to zero (see below).

The pattern of distribution of blood carbon dioxide is not well known in other vertebrates but it is probably essentially similar to that in man, with the formation of considerable amounts of labile carbamate and with bicarbonate accounting for the bulk of the non-labile fraction.

An interesting feature of the work on transitional forms is the apparent relationship between dependence on aerial respiration and the carbon dioxide combining and buffering capacity of the blood. This is particularly well exemplified by the lungfish sequence of Lenfant and Johansen, less well by their amphibian sequence (pp. 55, 129). Values for the relevant parameters are given in Table 12.3 in which some fishes and terrestrial vertebrates are included for

* In this context 'labile' means exchanged during the normal respiratory cycle.

Table 12.3 Carbon dioxide transport parameters for fully aquatic fish, transitional lungfish and amphibia and fully terrestrial mammals. Species in the transitional groups in order of increasing air-dependence. (From Lenfant et al.[139, 134])

	Arterial pCO_2 (mm)	Combined CO_2 at arterial pCO_2 (vols%)	Buffer capacity $\Delta HCO_3^-/\Delta pH$ (mM/l/pH)
Dogfish	2.3	6.8	—
Toadfish	3.5	7.5	—
Sea robin	3.5	8.5	—
Neoceratodus	3.6	11.2	13.3
Lepidosiren	7.0	21.0	14.9
Protopterus	25.7	43.0	15.2
Necturus	5.0	18.7	8.0
Amphiuma	7.0	36.0	9.2
R. catesbeiana	8.0	32.0	16.4
Platypus	28.0	41.0	—
Man	40.0	48.3	24.0

comparison. The superior buffering capacity of the blood of diving mammals has already been discussed (p. 166).

INVERTEBRATE CARBON DIOXIDE TRANSPORT

The situation in invertebrates has been closely studied only in a few cases, including some of the larger haemocyanin-bearing molluscs and arthropods and in the coelomic fluids of *Urechis* and *Sipunculus*. The same general principles seem to apply though the special relationship between plasma and corpuscles is usually absent. When respiratory pigments are present in solution they make up virtually the whole of the blood protein and the whole of the buffer capacity. If respiratory pigments are absent, small quantities of other blood proteins make up such buffer capacity as is present; in the absence of respiratory pigments little buffer capacity is required.

In *Limulus* carbon dioxide-binding capacity is directly proportional to haemocyanin content and weight for weight this pigment is as effective in buffering as haemoglobin. The buffer capacity is markedly influenced by the salt concentration of the solution, addition of 0.5M sodium chloride to pure haemocyanin solution increasing the capacity by 40%. *Limulus* blood which has a slight reversed Bohr effect fails to show any Haldane effect.[179]

A comparison of the bloods of *Busycon* and *Loligo* (Fig. 12.3) indicates that the specific carbon dioxide-carrying capacity of haemocyanin may be strikingly different from one animal to another. Although the carbon dioxide capacity of *Busycon* blood compares favourably with that of mammalian bloods and is more than twice that of *Loligo*, its oxygen capacity was only 1.6 vols % while that of

Loligo was 3.8 vols %. This discrepancy has not been explained. The very pronounced normal Bohr effect of *Loligo* blood is paralleled by its Haldane effect,
while the small reversed Bohr effect of *Busycon* is similarly matched.[176]

In the corpuscle-filled coelomic fluid of *Urechis* there is a situation analogous
to that of vertebrate blood. The buffer capacity of the coelomic fluid, which is
practically protein-free, is nil but the buffer power of the corpuscles (volume for
volume) is about one-fifth of the total in human blood; weight for weight the
two haemoglobins have very similar buffer values—about 0.17 mEq/g. At
physiological tensions the carbon dioxide content of *Urechis* coelomic fluid is
about equally divided between the 'plasma' and the corpuscles, while at higher
tensions the balance shifts in favour of the corpuscles. This suggests that carbonic
anhydrase is present in the corpuscles but that the chloride shift is limited. The

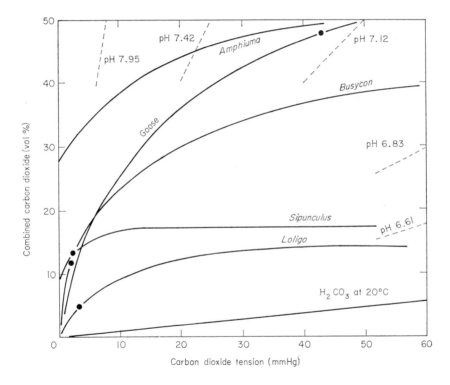

Fig. 12.3   Some representative carbon dioxide dissociation curves (combined gas only).
Busycon, Loligo and *Sipunculus* are typical of marine animals with low arterial pCO_2
(indicated by ●) while the goose is representative of lung-breathers with high arterial
pCO_2. The curve for *Amphiuma* is 'atypical', indicating a considerable amount of 'fixed'
carbon dioxide; such curves are found for a number of freshwater vertebrates. The
broken lines are the loci of the indicated pH values and are calculated from the Henderson-
Hasselbalch equation. (After Florkin[53])

coelomic fluid, which as we have seen earlier (p. 140) is probably more concerned with storage than with transport, exhibits neither Bohr nor Haldane effects.[177]

Carbamates and carbonic anhydrase in invertebrates

The possibility of carbamate formation has been investigated in a few invertebrates only, by a study of the time relations of carbon dioxide uptake *in vitro*. In the absence of carbonic anhydrase, bicarbonate formation is relatively slow, while carbon dioxide solution and carbamate formation are rapid. If the amount of carbon dioxide rapidly absorbed exceeds that which would be expected to dissolve, then carbamate formation is presumed. Such circumstantial evidence indicates that carbamate is not formed in the haemocyanins of *Octopus vulgaris*, *Helix pomatia*, *Homarus vulgaris* or *Cancer pagurus*, even though physical conditions in these bloods appear to be propitious.[233]

The distribution of carbonic anhydrase among invertebrates is better known. It is usually absent from the blood but has been found in the blood of *Lumbricus* and *Nereis* and in the coelomic fluids of *Sipunculus* and *Arenicola*. There are many records of the occurrence of this enzyme in gills including those of polychaetes, gastropods, cephalopods, lamellibranchs, *Limulus* and decapod crustacea and in the respiratory trees of holothurians.[70] In these situations the enzyme will presumably hasten the movement of bicarbonate out of the branchial blood. In a number of cases carbonic anhydrase has been detected in other tissues; these include muscles of *Loligo*, *Sepia*, *Murex* and *Limulus*, the body wall of various Anthozoa and the intestine of *Asterias* and *Holothuria*. Here the enzyme will presumably facilitate loading of blood with carbon dioxide. In the absence of blood corpuscles there seems to be no special reason for having carbonic anhydrase in the blood; indeed, if bicarbonate formation is to be encouraged there is every reason why this ion should migrate into a separate compartment (accompanied by cation or in exchange for anion) in order to be transported.

It should be noted that carbonic anhydrase occurs in many tissues (e.g. vertebrate kidney, pancreas, gastric mucosa etc.) where non-respiratory functions are presumed.[70]

CARBON DIOXIDE BINDING AND ADAPTATION

Although the diversity of established carbon dioxide dissociation curves does not match that of oxygen dissociation curves, there are reasonable grounds for supposing that the differences have some adaptive significance, as illustrated in Fig. 12.3. Of course, the curves lack the sigmoid character of many oxygen dissociation curves, there being nothing analogous to haem-haem interactions in the mechanisms of carbon dioxide-binding. This is of no consequence, since there is no reason for the pCO_2 buffer range to be adjusted to provide an adequate final diffusion gradient. It is, however, necessary for the curve to rise high enough to ensure a carbon dioxide capacity commensurate with oxygen capacity. All known curves do this with a handsome margin. It is also desirable that the curve should rise steeply to some point in excess of the normal venous pCO_2 tension so that all the labile carbon dioxide can be absorbed for a small change in pCO_2 and hence of pH. This point is also well satisfied in all cases.

Some carbon dioxide dissociation curves do not pass through the origin but indicate a substantial amount of 'fixed' or permanently bound carbon dioxide (Fig. 12.3). The conclusion is that there is insufficient weak acid in the blood to displace all the carbon dioxide present as bicarbonate even when the pCO_2 is reduced to zero. This is of no consequence for transport of respiratory carbon dioxide, since the non-fixed fraction exceeds the required turnover capacity but the significance of this fixed carbon dioxide is obscure. Such atypical dissociation curves have been found for a number of freshwater vertebrates (including *Rana catesbeana, Amphiuma tridactyla* and *Cyprinus carpio*)[53] and for *Helix pomatia*.[233] Unusually high carbon dioxide contents found in the bloods of various marine and freshwater invertebrates probably have a similar origin.[43]

I3   Conclusion

In such a broad field as animal respiration it is not possible to epitomize our knowledge and it is difficult to point broad generalizations. However, it is hoped that the selection of topics, treated with varying degrees of thoroughness in the preceding chapters, will serve to illustrate the complexity of factors and relationships which are involved in satisfying the needs of animals in a great diversity of situations.

The basic need is remarkably uniform. It is for the provision of oxygen, at a sufficient rate, to function as the final hydrogen acceptor in an apparently universal scheme of intracellular oxidation by electron transfer, which alone yields aerobically the energy for metabolic activities. This uniform need is served by an enormous diversity of arrangements for bringing the oxygen to the tissues and to a lesser extent for evacuating the resulting carbon dioxide. The reasons for this diversity are readily apparent. Increase in size and activity clearly depend on more 'efficient' methods of gas exchange and transport. These improvements though differing in detail from group to group may yet have important elements in common, e.g. counter-current flow of blood and respiratory medium; the adoption of closed circulatory systems. The characteristics of particular habitats or micro-habitats also impose certain conditions and limitations on gas exchange possibilities and so call forth a variety of adaptations.

Further, the adoption of certain modes of life, such as living in tubes or the diving of air-breathers, inevitably adds substantially to the need for adaptation towards the common goal. This feature, well illustrated by some of the examples which have been discussed at length, makes a thorough understanding of an animal's way of life essential for a proper interpretation of its adaptive properties and respiratory mechanisms. These adaptations and mechanisms form a vital part of the animal's homeostatic equipment and bear witness once again to the truth of Claude Bernard's celebrated aphorism (proposed as long ago as 1879): 'La fixité du milieu intérieur est la condition de la vie libre'.

Successful adaptations (we rarely see the unsuccessful ones) commonly involve morphological, physiological, behavioural and even purely chemical components. Sometimes these components may be regarded as independent but more often (at least in the final result) form an integrated whole. Such integration carries with it the dangers of inflexibility inherent in all highly specialized adaptations. However, there is one element in this picture which seems to have a peculiar potential for evolutionary variability, namely the properties of the respiratory pigment. If, as seems likely, all the more important functional properties of these molecules can be adjusted by normal processes of natural selection acting on the results of mutational changes in the protein replication machinery, then respiratory pigments form by far the most labile component in an integrated respiratory system. The course of evolution of air-breathing in vertebrates, for example, may be limited by pre-existing morphological features of the vascular system (p. 54) subject to the classical notion of irreversibility in evolution. The physico-chemical properties of the pigments, such as oxygen affinity, would by contrast seem subject to no such restrictions.

Such a view of the lability of respiratory pigments rests to a considerable extent on the belief that they are universally well adapted to the particular needs of the animals which possess them. The reader must form his own judgment on the adequacy of the case which has been made. In doing this he must bear in mind not only the frankly speculative nature of some of the interpretations (e.g. of reversed Bohr effects—p. 129) but also of the author's undoubted bias in regard to some of the apparently less speculative ones. Further work will be needed to clarify many of the questions which have been discussed and the incompleteness of the evidence on which one is tempted to base some generalizations must also be kept in mind.

While this work was in press many publications were added to the field, often bearing on the conclusions put forward here. Perutz,[244] for example, has proposed detailed models of the molecular mechanisms involved in haem-haem interactions, the Bohr effect and the functionally advantageous lowering of oxygen affinity by 2,3-diphosphoglycerate present in the erythrocytes. This strengthens the contention (p. 94) that X-ray diffraction and other studies of molecular structure would be critical for elucidating the functional properties of respiratory pigments.

On the other hand, our generalizations (p. 106) about the properties and role of haemocyanins in decapod crustacea must be re-examined in the light of a very careful study of respiration in the crab, *Cancer magister*. Here Johansen *et al*[241] have found a p50 of 19.6 mm at 10°C with arterial blood 99% saturated at 91 mm pO_2 and venous blood 50% saturated at 21 mm pO_2 (cf. Table 9.2 and Fig. 9.5). Since the highest oxygen affinity so far found in decapods is for a fresh water crayfish, *Procambarus simulans* with a p_{50} of 3.5 mm,[242, 243] this question should be investigated in relation to gill permeability and osmoregulation problems.

The author's own early work on the function of haemoglobin in *Nephtys* (pp. 135, 138) must also be reviewed following the recent investigation of the same species by Weber.[248] Here it seems I may have come to the right conclusion regarding the existence of an oxygen transfer system but for the wrong reasons.

Finally, the inevitably selective nature of this review must be re-emphasized. The conscientious reader will seek additional sources and the recent monograph by Steen[247] may be consulted with profit.

References

1. AKESTER, A. R. (1960). The comparative anatomy of the respiratory pathways in the domestic fowl (*Gallus domesticus*), pigeon (*Columba livia*) and domestic duck (*Anas platyrhyncha*). *J. Anat.*, **94**, 487–505.
2. ALBRITTON, E. C. ed. (1952). *Standard Values in Blood*. Saunders, Philadelphia and London.
3. ALEXANDER, R. MCN. (1967). *Functional Design in Fishes*. Hutchinson, London.
4. ANDERSEN, H. T. (1966). Physiological adaptations in diving vertebrates. *Physiol. Rev.*, **46**, 212–243.
5. ANTONINI, E. (1967). Hemoglobin and its reactions with ligands. *Science, N.Y.* **158**, 1417–1425.
6. BALDWIN, E. (1967). *Dynamic Aspects of Biochemistry*, 5th edn. University Press, Cambridge.
7. BANNISTER, R. G. (1960). The physiology of muscular exercise. In *The Structure and Function of Muscle*, Vol. 2, ed. G. H. Bourne. Academic Press, New York, and London.
8. BARBASHOVA, Z. I. (1964). Cellular level of adaptation. In *Adaptation to the Environment*. Sect. 4, Handbook of Physiology. ed. D. B. Dill. American Physiological Society, Washington.
9. BARCROFT, J. (1946). *Researches on Prenatal Life*. Blackwell, Oxford.
10. BARCROFT, J., ELLIOT, R. H. E., FLEXNER, L. B., HALL, F. G., HERKEL, W., MCCARTHY, E. F., MCCLURKIN, T. and TALAAT, M. (1934). Conditions of foetal circulation in the goat. *J. Physiol., Lond.* **83**, 192–214.
11. BARNES, T. C. (1937). *Textbook of General Physiology*. Blakiston, Philadelphia.
12. BARRON, D. H. and MESCHIA, G. (1954). A comparative study of the exchange of the respiratory gases across the placenta. *Cold Spring Harb. Symp. quant. Biol.*, **19**, 93–101.
13. BARTELS, H. (1964). Comparative physiology of oxygen transport in mammals. *Lancet*, 1964/II, 599–604.
14. BEADLE, L. C. and LIND, E. M. (1960). Research on the swamps of Uganda. *Uganda J.*, **24**, 84–98.
15. BĚLEHRÁDEK, J. (1935). *Temperature and Living Matter*. Protoplasma Monographien. Borntraeger, Berlin.
16. BENEDICT, F. G. (1938). *Vital Energetics. A Study in Comparative Basal Metabolism*. Publ. 503. Carnegie Inst. Washington D.C.
17. BENESCH, R. and BENESCH, R. E. (1964). Properties of haemoglobin H and their significance in relation to the function of haemoglobin. *Nature, Lond.*, **202**, 773–5.
18. BERG, K., JÓNASSON, P. M. and OCKELMANN, K. W. (1962). The respiration of some animals from the profundal zone of a lake. *Hydrobiologia*, **19**, 1–39.
19. BISHOP, D. W. (1950). Respiration and metabolism. In *Comparative Animal Physiology*, ed. C. L. Prosser. Saunders, Philadelphia and London.
20. BOCK, A. V., DILL, D. B., HURXTHAL, L. M., LAWRENCE, J. S., COOLIDGE, T. C., DAILEY, M. E. and HENDERSON, L. J. (1927). Blood as a physiochemical system. V. The composition and respiratory exchanges of normal human blood during work. *J. biol. Chem.*, **73**, 749–66.
21. BORDEN, M. A. (1931). A study of the respiration and of the function of haemo-

globin in *Planorbis corneus* and *Arenicola marina*. *J. mar. biol. Ass. U.K.*, **17**, 709–38.

22. BRAND, T. von. (1945). The anaerobic metabolism of invertebrates. *Biodynamica*, **5**, 165–284.

23. BRAND, T. von. (1946). *Anaerobiosis of Invertebrates*. Biodynamica Monograph No. 4. *Biodynamica*, Normandy, Mo.

24. BRODY, S. (1945). *Bioenergetics and Growth*. Reinhold, New York.

25. BURGER, J. W. and BRADLEY, S. E. (1951). The general form of circulation in the dogfish *Squalus acanthias*. *J. cell. comp. Physiol.*, **37**, 389–402.

26. BURGER, J. W. and SMYTHE, C. MCC. (1953). The general form of circulation in the lobster, *Homarus*. *J. cell. comp. Physiol.*, **42**, 369–83.

27. CARTER, G. S. (1955). *The Papyrus Swamps of Uganda*. Heffer, Cambridge.

28. CARTER, G. S. and BEADLE, L. C. (1930). The fauna of the swamps of the Paraguayan Chaco in relation to its environment. II. Respiratory adaptations in the fishes. *J. Linn. Soc. (Zool)*, **37**, 327–68.

29. CHANCE, B., COHEN, P., JOBSIS, F. and SCHOENER, B. (1962). Localized fluorometry of oxidation—reduction states of intracellular pyridine nucleotide in brain and kidney cortex of the anesthetized rat. *Science, N.Y.*, **136**, 325.

30. CLARK, R. B. (1956). The blood vascular system of *Nephtys* (Annelida, Polychaeta). *Q. Jl. Microsc. Sci.*, **97**, 235–49.

31. CLAUSEN, H. J. (1936). The effect of aggregation on the respiratory metabolism of the Brown Snake *Storeria dekayi*. *J. cell. comp. Physiol.*, **8**, 367–77.

32. COMROE, J. H. Jr. (1965). *Physiology of Respiration*. Year Book Medical Publishers, Chicago.

33. COMROE, J. H. Jr., FORSTER, R. E., DUBOIS, A. B., BRISCOE, W. A. and CARLSEN, E. (1962). *The Lung*, 2nd edn. Year Book Medical Publishers, Chicago.

34. CULLIS, A. F., MUIRHEAD, H., PERUTZ, M. F., ROSSMANN, M. G. and NORTH, A. C. T. (1962). The structure of haemoglobin. IX. A three-dimensional Fourier synthesis at 5.5 Å resolution: description of the structure. *Proc. R. Soc.*, A **265**, 161–87.

35. DALES, R. P. (1961). Observations on the respiration of the sabellid polychaete *Schizobranchia insignis*. *Biol. Bull. mar. biol. Lab., Woods Hole*, **121**, 82–91.

36. DAM, L. van. (1938). *On the Utilization of Oxygen and Regulation of Breathing in Some Aquatic Animals*. Thesis: Groningen.

37. DAUSEND, K. (1931). Über die Atmung der Tubificiden. *Z. vergl. Physiol.*, **14**, 557–608.

38. DICKERSON, R. E. and GEIS, I. (1969). *The Structure and Actions of Proteins*. Harper and Row, New York and London.

39. DILL, D. B., EDWARDS, H. T. and FLORKIN, M. (1932). Properties of the blood of the skate (*Raia ocellata*). *Biol. Bull. mar. biol. Lab., Woods Hole*, **62**, 23–36.

40. DÖBELN, W. von. (1956). Human standard and maximal metabolic rate in relation to fatfree body mass. *Acta physiol. scand.* **37**, Suppl. 126, 1–79.

41. DOLK, H. E. and POSTMA, N. (1927). Über die Haut- und Lungenatmung von *Rana temporaria*. *Z. vergl. Physiol.*, **5**, 417–44.

42. DUBOIS, E. F. (1936). *Basal Metabolism in Health and Disease*, 3rd edn. Lea & Febiger, Philadelphia.

43. DUVAL, M. and PORTIER, P. (1927). Sur la teneur en gaz carbonique total du sang des Invertébrés d'eau douce et des Invertébrés marins. *C.r. hebd. Séanc. Acad. Sci., Paris*, **184**, 1594–6.

44. ELSNER, R. (1969). Cardiovascular adjustments to diving. In *The Biology of Marine Mammals*. ed. H. T. Andersen, Academic Press, New York and London.

45. ELSNER, R., SHURLEY, J. T., HAMMOND, D. D. and BROOKS, R. E. (1970) Cerebral tolerance to hypoxemia in asphyxiated Weddell seals. *Respir. Physiol.*, **9**, 287–97.

46. EWER, D. W. (1959). A toad (*Xenopus laevis*) without haemoglobin. *Nature, Lond.*, **183**, 271.
47. EWER, R. F. (1942). On the function of haemoglobin in *Chironomus*. *J. exp. Biol.*, **18**, 197–205.
48. EWER, R. F. and FOX, H. M. (1940). On the function of chlorocruorin. *Proc. R. Soc.*, B**129**, 137–53.
49. FARBER, J. and RAHN, H. (1970). Gas exchange between air and water and the ventilation pattern in the electric eel. *Respir. Physiol.*, **9**, 151–61.
50. FARMANFARMAIAN, A. (1966). The respiratory physiology of echinoderms. In *Physiology of Echinodermata*, ed. R. A. Boolootian. Interscience, New York.
51. FLOREY, E. (1966). *An Introduction to General and Comparative Animal Physiology*. Saunders, Philadelphia and London.
52. FLORKIN, M. (1933). Recherches sur les hémérythrines. *Archs int. Physiol.*, **36**, 247–328.
53. FLORKIN, M. (1934). La fonction respiratoire du 'milieu intérieur' dans la série animale. *Annls Physiol. Physicochim. biol.*, **10**, 599–684.
54. FORSTER, R. E. (1964). Factors affecting the rate of exchange of oxygen between blood and tissues. In *Oxygen in the Animal Organism*. ed. F. Dickens and E. Neil. Pergamon, Oxford and London.
55. FOX, D. L. (1953). *Animal Biochromes and Structural Colours*. Cambridge University Press.
56. FOX, H. M. (1932). The oxygen affinity of chlorocruorin. *Proc. R. Soc.* B**111**, 356–63.
57. FOX, H. M. (1938). On the blood circulation and metabolism of sabellids. *Proc. R. Soc.*, B**125**, 554–69.
58. FOX, H. M. (1945). The oxygen affinity of certain invertebrate haemoglobins. *J. exp. Biol.* **21**, 161–65.
59. FOX, H. M. (1949). On chlorocruorin and haemoglobin. *Proc. R. Soc.*, B**136**, 378–88.
60. FOX, H. M. (1955). The effect of oxygen on the concentration of haem in invertebrates. *Proc. R. Soc.*, B**143**, 203–14.
61. FOX, H. M. and VEVERS, G. (1960). *The Nature of Animal Colours*. Sidgwick and Jackson, London.
62. FOX, H. M., WINGFIELD, C. A. and SIMMONDS, B. G. (1937). The oxygen consumption of ephemerid nymphs from flowing and from still waters in relation to the concentration of oxygen in the water. *J. exp. Biol.*, **14**, 210–18.
63. FOXON, G. E. H. (1964). Blood and Respiration. In *Physiology of the Amphibia*, ed. J. A. Moore. Academic Press, New York and London.
64. FRY, F. E. J. and HART, J. S. (1948). The relation of temperature to oxygen consumption in the goldfish. *Biol. Bull. mar. biol. Lab., Woods Hole*, **94**, 66–77.
65. FÜSSER, H. and KRÜGER, F. (1951). Vergleichende Versuche zur Atmungsphysiologie von *Planorbis corneus* und *Limnaea stagnalis* (Gastropoda, Pulmonata). *Z. vergl. Physiol.*, **33**, 14–52.
66. GAHLENBECK, H. and BARTELS, H. (1970). Blood gas transport properties in gill and lung forms of the axolotl (*Amblystoma mexicanum*). *Respir. Physiol.*, **9**, 175–182.
67. GANS, C. and HUGHES, G. M. (1967). The mechanism of lung ventilation in the tortoise *Testudo graeca* Linné. *J. exp. Biol.*, **47**, 1–20.
68. GHIRETTI, F. (1966). Respiration. In *Physiology of Mollusca*, Vol. 2. ed. K. M. Wilbur and C. M. Yonge. Academic Press, New York and London.
69. GILCHRIST, B. M. (1954). Haemoglobin in *Artemia*. *Proc. R. Soc.*, B**143**, 136–46.
70. GOOR, H. van (1948). Carbonic anhydrase, its properties, distribution and significance for carbon transport. *Enzymologia*, **13**, 73–164.
71. GRAY, I. E. (1957). A comparative study of the gill areas of crabs. *Biol. Bull. mar. biol. Lab., Woods Hole*, **112**, 34–42.

72. GREGERSEN, M. I. and RAWSON, R. A. (1959). Blood Volume. *Physiol. Rev.*, **39**, 307–42.
73. HALDANE, J. S. (1922). *Respiration.* Yale University Press, New Haven.
74. HALL, F. G. (1929). The influence of varying oxygen tensions upon the rate of oxygen consumption in the blood. *Am. J. Physiol.*, **88**, 212–18.
75. HALL, F. G., DILL, D. B. and BARRON, E. S. G. (1936). Comparative physiology in high altitudes. *J. cell. comp. Physiol.*, **8**, 301–13.
76. HALL, V. E. (1931). Muscular activity and oxygen consumption of *Urechis caupo*. *Biol. Bull. mar. biol. Lab.*, *Woods Hole*, **61**, 400–16.
77. HAUGHTON, T. M., KERKUT, G. A. and MUNDAY, K. A. (1958). The oxygen dissociation and alkaline denaturation of haemoglobins from two species of earthworms. *J. exp. Biol.* **35**, 360–8.
78. HAZELHOFF, E. H. (1938). Über die Ausnützung des Sauerstoffs bei verschiedenen Wassertieren. *Z. vergl. Physiol.*, **26**, 306–27.
79. HAZELHOFF, E. H. (1951). Structure and function of the lung of birds. *Poult. Sci.*, **30**, 3–10.
80. HEILBRUNN, L. V. (1943). *An Outline of General Physiology*, 2nd edn. Saunders, Philadelphia and London.
81. HEMMINGSEN, A. M. (1950). The relation of standard (basal) energy metabolism to total fresh weight of living organisms. *Rep. Steno meml Hosp.*, **4**, 7–58.
82. HEMMINGSEN, A. M. (1960). Energy metabolism as related to body size and respiratory surfaces, and its evolution. *Rep. Steno meml Hosp.*, **9**, 1–110.
83. HEMMINGSEN, E. H. (1965). Accelerated transfer of oxygen through solutions of heme compounds. *Acta physiol. scand.*, **64**, Suppl. 246, 1–53.
84. HEMMINGSEN, E. and SCHOLANDER, P. F. (1960). Specific transport of oxygen through hemoglobin solutions. *Science, N.Y.*, **132**, 1379–81.
85. HENDERSON, L. J. (1928). *Blood; a Study in General Physiology.* Yale University Press, New Haven.
86. HILL, R. B. and WELSH, J. H. (1966). Heart, circulation and blood cells. In *Physiology of Mollusca*, Vol. 2. ed. K. M. Wilbur and C. M. Yonge. Academic Press, New York and London.
87. HILLS, B. A. and HUGHES, G. M. (1970). A dimensional analysis of oxygen transfer in the fish gill. *Respir. Physiol.*, **9**, 126–40.
88. HUGHES, G. M. (1961). How a fish extracts oxygen from water. *New Scientist*, **11**, 346–8.
89. HUGHES, G. M. (1963). *Comparative Physiology of Vertebrate Respiration.* Heinemann, London.
90. HUGHES, G. M. (1964). Fish respiratory homeostasis. *Symp. Soc. exp. Biol.*, **18**, 81–107.
91. HUGHES, G. M., KNIGHTS, B. and SCAMMELL, C. A. (1969). The distribution of pO_2 and hydrostatic pressure changes within the branchial chambers in relation to gill ventilation of the shore crab, *Carcinus maenas* L. *J. exp. Biol.*, **51**, 203–20.
92. HUGHES, G. M. and SHELTON, G. (1958). The mechanism of gill ventilation in three fresh water teleosts. *J. exp. Biol.*, **35**, 807–23.
93. HUGHES, G. M. and SHELTON, G. (1962). Respiratory mechanisms and their nervous control in fish. In *Advances in Comparative Physiology and Biochemistry*, Vol. 1. ed. O. Lowenstein. Academic Press, New York and London.
94. HUNTER, W. R. (1953). The condition of the mantle cavity in two pulmonate snails living in Loch Lomond. *Proc. R. Soc. Edinb.*, B**65**, 143–65.
95. HURTADO, A. (1964). Animals in high altitudes: resident man. In *Adaptation to the Environment*. Sect. 4, Handbook of Physiology. ed. D. B. Dill. American Physiological Society, Washington.
96. HUTCHINSON, V. H., WHITFORD, W. G. and KOHL, M. (1968). Relation of body size and surface area to gas exchange in Anurans. *Physiol. Zoöl.* **41**, 65–85.
97. IRVING, L. (1964). Comparative anatomy and physiology of gas transport

mechanisms. In *Respiration*, Vol. 1, eds. W. O. Fenn and H. Rahn. Handbook of Physiology, Sect. 3, American Physiological Society, Washington, D.C.

98. JEUKEN, M. (1957). *A Study of the Respiration of* Misgurnus fossilis (L.), *the pond loach*. Thesis. Leiden.

99. JOHANSEN, K., HANSON, D. and LENFANT, C. (1970). Respiration in a primitive air breather, *Amia calva. Respir. Physiol.*, **9**, 162–74.

100. JOHANSEN, K. and LENFANT, C. (1967). Respiratory function in the South American Lungfish, *Lepidosiren paradoxa. J. exp. Biol.*, **46**, 205–18.

101. JOHANSEN, K. and LENFANT, C. (1968). Respiration in the African lungfish *Protopterus aethiopicus*. II. Control of breathing. *J. exp. Biol.*, **49**, 453–68.

102. JOHANSEN, K. and MARTIN, A. W. (1962). Circulation in the cephalopod *Octopus dofleini. Comp. Biochem. Physiol.*, **5**, 161–76.

103. JOHANSEN, K. and MARTIN, A. W. (1966). Circulation in a giant earthworm, *Glossoscolex giganteus*. II. Respiratory properties of blood and some patterns of gas exchange. *J. exp. Biol.*, **45**, 165–72.

104. JOHNSON, M. L. (1942). The respiratory function of the haemoglobin of the earthworm. *J. exp. Biol.*, **18**, 266–77.

105. JONES, J. D. (1955). Observations on the respiratory physiology and on the haemoglobin of the polychaete genus *Nephthys*, with special reference to *N. hombergii*. (Aud et M. Edw.). *J. exp. Biol.*, **32**, 110–25.

106. JONES, J. D. (1961). Aspects of respiration in *Planorbis corneus* L. and *Lymnaea stagnalis* (Gastropoda, Pulmonata). *Comp. Biochem. Physiol.*, **4**, 1–29.

107. JONES, J. D. (1963). The functions of the respiratory pigments of invertebrates. In *Problems in Biology*, Vol. 1. ed. G. A. Kerkut. Pergamon, Oxford and New York.

108. JONES, J. D. (1964a). The role of haemoglobin in the aquatic pulmonate, *Planorbis corneus. Comp. Biochem. Physiol.*, **12**, 283–95.

109. JONES, J. D. (1964b). Respiratory gas exchange in the aquatic pulmonate, *Biomphalaria sudanica. Comp. Biochem. Physiol.*, **12**, 297–310.

110. JONES, J. D. The role of haemocyanin in the pulmonate gastropod *Lymnaea stagnalis*. (in preparation).

111. DE JONGH, H. J. and GANS, C. (1969). On the mechanism of respiration in the bullfrog, *Rana catesbeiana*: A reassessment. *J. Morph.*, **127**, 259–90.

112. JORDAN, H. J. (1930). Le réglage de la consommation de l'oxygène chez les animaux à 'tension gazeuse alvéolaire inconstante.' *Archs néerl. Physiol.*, **15**, 198–212.

113. KAO, F. F. (1963) An experimental study of the pathways involved in exercise hyperpnoea employing cross-circulation techniques. In *The Regulation of Human Respiration*, ed. D. J. C. Cunningham and B. B. Lloyd. Blackwell, Oxford.

114. KAYSER, C. H. (1950). Le problème de la loi des tailles et de la loi des surfaces tel qu'il apparaît dans l'étude de la calorification des batrachiens et reptiles et des mammifères hibernants. *Archs Sci. physiol.*, **4**, 361–78.

115. KELLOG, R. H. (1963). The role of carbon dioxide in altitude acclimatization. In *The Regulation of Human Respiration*, ed. D. J. C. Cunningham and B. B. Lloyd. Blackwell, Oxford.

116. KENDREW, J. C., DICKERSON, R. E., STRANDBERG, B. E., HART, R. G., DAVIES, D. R., PHILLIPS, D. C. and SHORE, V. C. (1960). Structure of myoglobin. A three dimensional Fourier synthesis at 2 Å resolution. *Nature, Lond.*, **185**, 422–427.

117. KLEIBER, M. (1941). Body size and metabolism of liver slices *in vitro*. *Proc. Soc. exp. Biol. Med.*, **48**, 419–22.

118. KLOTZ, I. M. and KLOTZ, T. A. (1955). Oxygen carrying proteins: a comparison of the oxygenation reaction in hemocyanin and hemerythrin with that in hemoglobin. *Science, N.Y.*, **121**, 477–80.

119. KREBS, A. H. (1950). Body size and tissue respiration. *Biochim. biophys. Acta*, **4**, 249–69.
120. KREUZER, F. (1970). Facilitated diffusion of oxygen and its possible significance; a review. *Respir. Physiol.*, **9**, 1–30.
121. KRIEBEL, M. E. (1963). Effect of blood pressure on the isolated tunicate heart. *Biol. Bull. mar. biol. Lab.*, *Woods Hole*, **125**, 358.
122. KROGH, A. (1904). On the cutaneous and pulmonary respiration of the frog. *Skand. Arch. Physiol.*, **15**, 328–419.
123. KROGH, A. (1916). *The Respiratory Exchange of Animals and Man*. Longmans, Green, London.
124. KROGH, A. (1919a). The rate of diffusion of gases through animal tissues, with some remarks on the coefficient of invasion. *J. Physiol.*, *Lond.*, **52**, 391–408.
125. KROGH, A. (1919b). The supply of oxygen to the tissues and the regulation of the capillary circulation. *J. Physiol.*, *Lond.*, **52**, 457–74.
126. KROGH, A. (1920) Studien über Tracheenrespiration II. Über Gasdiffusion in den Tracheen. *Pflügers Arch. ges. Physiol.*, **179**, 95–112.
127. KROGH, A. (1929). *The Anatomy and Physiology of Capillaries*. Yale University Press, New Haven. Reprinted 1959, Hafner, New York.
128. KROGH, A. (1941). *The Comparative Physiology of Respiratory Mechanisms*. University of Pennsylvania Press, Philadelphia.
129. KROGH, M. (1915). The diffusion of gases through the lungs of man. *J. Physiol.*, *Lond.*, **49**, 271–300.
130. KUHN, W., RAMEL, A., KUHN, H. J. and MARTI, E. (1963). The filling mechanism of the swimbladder. *Experientia*, **19**, 497–511.
131. LANGLEY, L. L. (1949). Respiration of the electric eel. *Am. J. Physiol.*, **159**, 578.
132. LANKESTER, E. R. (1869). Spectroscopic examination of certain animal substances. *J. Anat.*, **4**, 119.
133. LARIMER, J. L. (1959). Gas transport of mammalian blood as related to size. *Fedn Proc. Fedn Am. Socs exp. Biol.*, **18**, 87.
134. LEE, D. L. and SMITH, M. H. (1965). Hemoglobins of parasitic animals. *Expl. Parasit.*, **16**, 392–424.
135. LEHMANN, H. and HUNTSMAN, R. G. (1961). Why are red cells the shape they are? The evolution of the human red cell. In *Functions of the Blood*, ed. R. G. Macfarlane and A. H. T. Robb-Smith. Blackwell, Oxford.
136. LEITCH, I. (1916) The function of haemoglobin in invertebrates with special reference to *Planorbis* and *Chironomus* larvae. *J. Physiol.*, *Lond.*, **50**, 370–9.
137. LENFANT, C. (1969). Physiological properties of blood of marine mammals. In *The Biology of Marine Mammals*, ed. H. T. Andersen. Academic Press, New York and London.
138. LENFANT, C. and JOHANSEN, K. (1967). Respiratory adaptations in selected amphibians. *Respir. Physiol.*, **2**, 247–60.
139. LENFANT, C. and JOHANSEN, K. (1968). Respiration in the African lungfish *Protopterus aethiopicus*. I. Respiratory properties of blood and normal patterns of breathing and gas exchange. *J. exp. Biol.*, **49**, 437–52.
140. LENFANT, C., JOHANSEN, K. and GRIGG, G. C. (1966/67). Respiratory properties of blood and pattern of gas exchange in the lungfish *Neoceratodus forsteri* (Krefft). *Respir. Physiol.*, **2**, 1–21.
141. LENFANT, C., JOHANSEN, K. and TORRANCE, J. D. (1970). Gas transport and oxygen storage capacity in some pinnipeds and the sea otter. *Respir. Physiol.*, **9**, 277–86.
142. LEVY, R. I. and SCHNEIDERMAN, H. A. (1958). An experimental solution to the paradox of discontinuous respiration in insects. *Nature*, *Lond.*, **182**, 491–3.
143. LOCKWOOD, A. P. M. (1968). *Aspects of the Physiology of Crustacea*. Oliver and Boyd, Edinburgh.

144. LONGMUIR, I. S. (1966). Tissue respiration. In *Advances in Respiratory Physiology*, ed. C. G. Caro. Edward Arnold, London.
145. MANWELL, C. (1958). The oxygen-respiratory pigment equilibrium of the hemocyanin and myoglobin of the amphineuran mollusc *Cryptochiton stellari. J. cell. comp. Physiol.*, **52**, 341–52.
146. MANWELL, C. (1959). Alkaline denaturation and oxygen equilibrium of annelid hemoglobins. *J. cell. comp. Physiol.*, **53**, 61–74.
147. MANWELL, C. (1960). Comparative physiology: Blood pigments. *A. Rev. Physiol.*, **22**, 191–244.
148. MANWELL, C. (1963). The blood proteins of cyclostomes. A study in phylogenetic and ontogenetic biochemistry. In *The Biology of Myxine*, ed. A. Brodal and R. Fange. Universitetsforlaget, Oslo.
149. MANWELL, C. (1964). Chemistry, genetics and function of invertebrate respiratory pigments—Configurational changes and allosteric effects. In *Oxygen in the Animal Organism*, ed. F. Dickens and E. Neil. Pergamon, Oxford and New York.
150. MANWELL, C., SOUTHWARD, E. C. and SOUTHWARD, A. J. (1966). Preliminary studies on haemoglobin and other proteins of the Pogonophora. *J. mar. biol. Ass. U.K.*, **46**, 115–24.
151. MARTIN, A. W. and FUHRMAN, F. (1955). Relationship between summated tissue respiration and metabolic rate in the mouse and dog. *Physiol. Zoöl.*, **28**, 18–34.
152. MARTIN, A. W. and JOHANSEN, K. (1965). Adaptations of the circulation of invertebrate animals. In *Circulation*, Vol. 3, ed. W. F. Hamilton and P. Dow, Sect. 2, Handbook of Physiology, American Physiological Society, Washington D.C.
153. MCCUTCHEON, F. H. (1938). The oxygen affinity of haemoglobin in splenectomised bullfrogs. *J. exp. Biol.*, **15**, 431–436.
154. MCMAHON, B. R. (1969). A functional analysis of the aquatic and aerial respiratory movements of an African lungfish, *Protopterus aethiopicus*, with reference to the evolution of the lung-ventilation mechanism in vertebrates. *J. exp. Biol.*, **51**, 407–30.
155. MILLAR, R. H. (1953). Ciona. *L.M.B.C. Mem. typ. Br. mar. Pl. Anim.*, **35**, 1–123.
156. MILLER, P. L. (1964). Respiration—Aerial gas transport. In *Physiology of Insecta*, Vol. 3, ed. M. Rockstein. Academic Press, New York and London.
157. MITCHELL, R. A. (1966). Cerebrospinal fluid and the regulation of respiration. In *Advances in Respiratory Physiology*, ed. C. G. Caro. Edward Arnold, London.
158. MOREHOUSE, L. E. and MILLER, A. T. (1963). *Physiology of Exercise*. C. V. Mosby Co., Saint Louis.
159. MORTON, J. E. and YONGE, C. M. (1964). Classification and structure of mollusca. In *Physiology of Mollusca*, Vol. 1, ed. K. M. Wilbur and C. M. Yonge. Academic Press, New York and London.
160. MOSSMAN, H. W. (1937). Comparative morphogenesis of the fetal membranes and accessory uterine structures. *Carnegie Inst. Contr. Embryol.* **26**, 129–246.
161. NIELSEN, M. and ASMUSSEN, E. (1963). Humoral and nervous control of breathing in exercise. In *The Regulation of Human Respiration*, ed. D. J. C. Cunningham and B. B. Lloyd. Blackwell, Oxford.
162. OTIS, A. B. (1963). The control of respiratory gas exchange between blood and tissues. In *The Regulation of Human Respiration*, ed. D. J. C. Cunningham and B. B. Lloyd. Blackwell, Oxford.
163. PARER, J. T. (1970). Oxygen transport in human subjects with hemoglobin variants having altered oxygen affinity. *Respir. Physiol.*, **9**, 43–9.
164. PATTLE, R. E. (1965). Surface lining of lung alveoli. *Physiol. Rev.*, **45**, 48–79.

165. PATTLE, R. E. (1969). The development of the foetal lung. In *Foetal Autonomy*, ed. G. E. W. Wolstenholme and M. O'Connor. Churchill, London.
166. PEARSE, A. D. (1929). The migrations of animals from sea to land. *Carnegie. Inst. Tortugas Papers*, **391**, 205–23.
167. PEARSE, A. S. (1936). *The Migrations of Animals from Sea to Land*. Duke University Press, Durham, N.C.
168. PEARSON, O. P. (1950). The metabolism of humming birds. *Condor*, **52**, 145–52.
169. PERUTZ, M. F. (1964). The haemoglobin molecule. *Scient. Am.*, **211**, 64–76.
170. PORTMANN, A. (1950). Les organes respiratoires. In *Traité de Zoologie*, Vol. 15, ed. P.-P. Grassé. Masson, Paris.
171. PROBST, G. (1933). Über den Sauerstoffverbrauch in der Lunge von *Planorbis corneus* und *Limnaea stagnalis* und die Bedeutung des Hämoglobins für die Lungenatmung von *Planorbis*. *Verh. naturf. Ges. Basel*, **114**, 386–7.
172. PROSSER, C. L. (1950). Circulation of body fluids. In *Comparative Animal Physiology*, 1st edn., ed. C. L. Prosser. Saunders, Philadelphia and London.
173. PROSSER, C. L. (1961a). Circulation of body fluids. In *Comparative Animal Physiology*, 2nd edn., ed. C. L. Prosser and F. A. Brown, Jr. Saunders, Philadelphia and London.
174. PROSSER, C. L. (1961b). Oxygen: respiration and metabolism. In *Comparative Animal Physiology*, 2nd edn., ed. C. L. Prosser and F. A. Brown, Jr. Saunders, Philadelphia and London.
175. PROSSER, C. L. (1961c). Respiratory functions of body fluids. In *Comparative Animal Physiology*, 2nd edn., ed. C. L. Prosser and F. A. Brown, Jr. Saunders, Philadelphia and London.
176. REDFIELD, A. C., COOLIDGE, T. and HURD, A. L. (1926). The transport of oxygen and carbon dioxide by some bloods containing hemocyanin. *J. biol. Chem.* **69**, 475–509.
177. REDFIELD, A. C. and FLORKIN, M. (1931). The respiratory function of the blood of *Urechis caupo*. *Biol. Bull. mar. biol. Lab., Woods Hole*, **61**, 185–210.
178. REDFIELD, A. C. and GOODKIND, R. (1929). The significance of the Bohr effect in the respiration and asphyxiation of the squid *Loligo pealei*. *J. exp. Biol.*, **6**, 340–9.
179. REDFIELD, A. C., HUMPHREYS, G. and INGALLS, E. N. (1929). The respiratory proteins of the blood IV. The buffer action of the hemocyanin in the blood of *Limulus polyphemus*. *J. biol. Chem.*, **82**, 759–73.
180. REDMOND, J. R. (1955). The respiratory function of hemocyanin in crustacea. *J. cell. comp. Physiol.*, **46**, 209–47.
181. REDMOND, J. R. (1962). Oxygen-hemocyanin relationships in the land crab *Cardisoma guanhumi*. *Biol. Bull. mar. biol. Lab., Woods Hole*, **122**, 252–62.
182. REDMOND, J. R. (1968). The respiratory function of hemocyanin. In *Physiology and Biochemistry of Haemocyanins*, ed. F. Ghiretti. Academic Press, New York and London.
183. REDMOND, J. R. (1968). Transport of oxygen by the blood of the land crab, *Gecarcinus lateralis*. *Am. Zool.* **8**, 471–9.
184. RIGGS, A. (1941). The metamorphosis of hemoglobin in the bullfrog. *J. gen. Physiol.*, **35**, 23–40.
185. RIGGS, A. (1960). Nature and significance of the Bohr effect in mammalian hemoglobins. *J. gen. Physiol.*, **43**, 737–52.
186. RIGGS, A. (1965). Functional properties of hemoglobins. *Physiol. Rev.*, **45**, 619–73.
187. ROCCA, E. and GHIRETTI, F. (1963). Ricerche sulle Emocianine. VII. Sulla capacità dell'emocianine di *Octopus vulgaris* di legare l'ossido di carbonio. *Boll. Soc. ital. Biol. sper.*, **39**, 2075–7.

G

188. ROOT, R. W. (1934). The combination of carbon monoxide with hemoglobin. *J. biol. Chem.*, **104**, 239–44.

189. RUBNER, M. (1883). Über den Einfluss der Körpergrösse auf Stoff- und Kraftwechsel. *Z. Biol.*, **19**, 535–62.

190. RUITER, L. DE, WOLVEKAMP, H. P., van TOOREN, A. J. and VLASBLOM, A. (1952). Experiments on the efficiency of the 'physical gill' (*Hydrous piceus* L., *Naucoris cimicoides* L. and *Notonecta glauca* L.). *Acta physiol. pharmacol. néerl.*, **2**, 180–213.

191. RUSHMER, R. F. (1961). *Cardiovascular Dynamics*, 2nd edn. Saunders, Philadelphia and London.

192. RUUD, J. T. (1954). Vertebrates without erythrocytes and blood pigment. *Nature, Lond.*, **173**, 848–50.

193. SALT, G. W. and ZEUTHEN, E. (1960). The respiratory system. In *Biology and Comparative Physiology of Birds*, Vol. 1, ed. A. J. Marshall. Academic Press, New York and London.

194. SAUNDERS, R. L. (1961). The irrigation of the gills in fishes. I. Studies of the mechanism of branchial irrigation. *Can. J. Physiol.*, **39**, 637–53.

195. SCHMIDT-NIELSEN, B., SCHMIDT-NIELSEN, K., HOUPT, T. R. and JARNUM, S. A. (1956). Water balance of the camel. *Am. J. Physiol.*, **185**, 185–94.

196. SCHMIDT-NIELSEN, K., HAINSWORTH, F. R. and MURRISH, D. E. (1970). Countercurrent heat exchange in the respiratory passages: Effect on water and heat balance. *Respir. Physiol.*, **9**, 263–76.

197. SCHMIDT-NIELSEN, K. and LARIMER, J. P. (1958). Oxygen dissociation curves of mammalian blood in relation to body size. *Am. J. Physiol.*, **195**, 424–8.

198. SCHMIDT-NIELSEN, K. and PENNYCUIK, P. (1961). Capillary density in mammals in relation to body size and oxygen consumption. *Am. J. Physiol.*, **200**, 746–50.

199. SCHOLANDER, P. F. (1940). Experimental investigations on the respiratory function in diving mammals and birds. *Hvalråd. Skr.*, **22**, 1–131.

200. SCHOLANDER, P. F. (1957). The wonderful net. *Scient. Am.* April 1957, 97–107.

201. SCHOLANDER, P. F. (1960). Oxygen transport through hemoglobin solutions. *Science, N.Y.*, **131**, 585–90.

202. SHEPARD, M. P. (1955). Resistance and tolerance of young speckled trout (*Salvelinus fontinalis*) to oxygen lack with special reference to low oxygen acclimation. *J. Fish. Res. Bd Can.*, **12**, 387–446.

203. SPOEK, G. L. (1962). Verslag van onderzoekingen gedaan in het Stazione Zoologica te Napels. *Kon. Ned. Akad. Wet., Versl. Afd. Natuurk.* **71**, 29–35.

204. SPOEK, G. L., BAKKER, H. and WOLVEKAMP, H. P. (1964). Experiments on the haemocyanin-oxygen equilibrium of the blood of the edible snail (*Helix pomatia* L.). *Comp. Biochem. Physiol.*, **12**, 209–21.

205. STEPHENSON, J. (1930). *The Oligochaeta*. Oxford University Press, London.

206. STICKNEY, J. C. and van LIERE, E. J. (1953). Acclimatization to low oxygen tension. *Physiol. Rev.*, **33**, 13–34.

207. STURKIE, P. D. (1954). *Avian Physiology*. Comstock, Ithaca.

208. TENNEY, S. M. and TENNEY, J. B. (1970). Quantitative morphology of cold-blooded lungs: amphibia and reptilia. *Respir. Physiol.*, **9**, 197–215.

209. TERWILLIGER, R. C. and READ, K. R. H. (1969). Quaternary structure of the radular muscle myoglobin of the gastropod mollusc *Buccinum undatum* L. *Comp. Biochem. Physiol.*, **31**, 55–64.

210. THOMAS, H. J. (1954). The oxygen uptake of the lobster (*Homarus vulgaris* Edw.). *J. exp. Biol.*, **31**, 228–51.

211. THORPE, W. H. (1950). Plastron respiration in aquatic insects. *Biol. Rev.*, **25**, 344–91.

212. VERNBERG, F. J. (1954). The respiratory metabolism of marine teleosts in relation to activity and body size. *Biol. Bull. mar. biol. Lab., Woods Hole*, **106**, 360–70.

213. WALD, G. (1952). Biochemical evolution. In *Modern Trends in Physiology and Biochemistry*, ed. E. S. G. Barron. Academic Press, New York and London.
214. WALD, G. and ALLEN, D. W. (1957). The equilibrium between cytochrome oxidase and carbon monoxide. *J. gen. Physiol.*, **40**, 593–608.
215. WALSHE, B. M. (1950). The function of haemoglobin in *Chironomus plumosus* under natural conditions. *J. exp. Biol.*, **27**, 73–95.
216. WALSHE-MAETZ, B. M. (1952). Environment and respiratory control in certain crustacea. *Nature, Lond.*, **169**, 750–1.
217. WALSHE-MAETZ, B. M. (1953). Le métabolisme de *Chironomus plumosus* dans des conditions naturelles. *Physiologia comp. Oecol.*, **3**, 135–54.
218. WASTL, H. (1928). Beobachtungen über die Blutgase des Karpfenblutes. *Biochem. Z.*, **197**, 363–80.
219. WASTL, H. and LEINER, G. (1931a). Beobachtungen über die Blutgase bei Vögeln I. *Pflügers Arch. ges. Physiol.*, **227**, 368–420.
220. WASTL, H. and LEINER, G. (1931b). Beobachtungen über die Blutgase bei Vögeln II. *Pflügers Arch. ges. Physiol.*, **227**, 421–59.
221. WEBER, R. E. (1963). Aspects of haemoglobin function in the larvae of the midge, *Chironomus plumosus* L. *Proc. K. ned. Akad. Wet.*, C **66**, 284–95.
222. WELLS, G. P. (1949a). The respiratory movements of *Arenicola marina* L.; intermittent irrigation of the tube and intermittent aerial respiration. *J. mar. biol. Ass. U.K.* **28**, 447–64.
223. WELLS, G. P. (1949b). The behaviour of *Arenicola marina* L. in sand and the role of spontaneous activity cycles. *J. mar. biol. Ass. U.K.*, **28**, 465–78.
224. WELLS, G. P. (1951). On the behaviour of *Sabella*. *Proc. R. Soc.*, B **138**, 278–99.
225. WELLS, G. P. (1952). The respiratory significance of the crown in the polychaete worms *Sabella* and *Myxicola*. *Proc. R. Soc.*, B **140**, 70–82.
226. WIGGLESWORTH, sir V. B. (1965). *The Principles of Insect Physiology*, 6th edn. Methuen, London.
227. WINTERSTEIN, H. (1909). Zur Kenntnis der Blutgase wirbelloser Seetiere. *Biochem. Z.* **19**, 384–424.
228. WINTERSTEIN, H. (1925). Über die chemische Regulierung der Atmung bei den Cephalopoden. *Z. vergl. Physiol.*, **2**, 315–328.
229. WITTENBERG, J. B. (1963). Facilitated diffusion of oxygen through haemerythrin solution. *Nature, Lond.*, **199**, 816–7.
230. WITTENBERG, J. B., SCHWEND, M. J. and WITTENBERG, B. A. (1964). The secretion of oxygen into the swim-bladder of fish. III. The role of carbon dioxide. *J. gen. Physiol.*, **48**, 337–55.
231. WOLVEKAMP, H. P. (1949). Oxygen and carbon dioxide transport by blood containing haemocyanin. In *Haemoglobin: A Symposium in Memory of Sir Joseph Barcroft*, ed. F. J. W. Roughton. Butterworth, London.
232. WOLVEKAMP, H. P. (1955). Die physikalische Kieme der Wasserinsekten. *Experientia*, **11**, 294–301.
233. WOLVEKAMP, H. P. (1961). The evolution of oxygen transport. In *Functions of the Blood*, ed. R. G. Macfarlane and A. H. T. Robb-Smith. Blackwell, Oxford.
234. WOLVEKAMP, H. P. and VREEDE, M. C. (1941). On the gas binding properties of the blood of the lugworm (*Arenicola marina* L.). *Archs néerl. Physiol.*, **25**, 265–76.
235. WOOD, D. W. (1968). *Principles of Animal Physiology* Edward Arnold, London.
236. YONGE, C. M. (1947). The pallial organs in the Aspidobranch Gastropoda and their evolution throughout the Mollusca. *Phil. Trans. R. Soc.*, B **232**, 443–518.
237. ZAAIJER, J. J. P. and WOLVEKAMP, H. P. (1958). Some experiments on the haemoglobin-oxygen equilibrium in the blood of the ramshorn (*Planorbis corneus* L). *Acta physiol. pharmac. néerl.*, **7**, 56–77.

238. ZEUTHEN, E. (1953). Oxygen uptake as related to body size in organisms. *Q. Rev. Biol.*, **28**, 1–12.
239. ZEUTHEN, E. (1955). Comparative physiology (respiration). *A. Rev. Physiol.*, **17**, 459–82.
240. ZUCKERKANDL, E. (1957). La teneur en oxygène de l'hémolymphe artérielle de *Maia squinado* aux divers stades d'intermue. *C.r. Séanc. Soc. Biol.*, **151**, 524–8.

Added in press

241. JOHANSEN, K., LENFANT, C. and MECKLENBURG, T. A. (1970). Respiration in the crab, *Cancer magister*. *Z. vergl. Physiol.*, **70**, 1–19.
242. LARIMER, J. L. (1964). The patterns of diffusion across crustacean gill membranes. *J. cell. comp. Physiol.*, **64**, 139–48.
243. LARIMER, J. L. and GOLD, A. H. (1961). The responses of the crayfish, *Procambarus simulans*, to respiratory stress. *Physiol. Zool.*, **34**, 167–76.
244. PERUTZ, M. F. (1970). Stereochemistry of cooperative effects in haemoglobin. *Nature, Lond.*, **228**, 726–39.
245. PERUTZ, M. F., ROSSMANN, M. G., CULLIS, A. F., MUIRHEAD, H., WILL, G. and NORTH, A. C. T. (1960). Structure of haemoglobin. A three-dimensional Fourier synthesis at 5.5 Å resolution, obtained by X-ray analysis. *Nature, Lond.*, **185**, 416–22.
246. ROUGHTON, F. J. W. (1964). Transport of oxygen and carbon dioxide. In *Respiration*, Vol. 1, ed. W. O. Fenn and H. Rahn, Sect. 3, Handbook of Physiology, American Physiological Society, Washington D.C.
247. STEEN, J. B. (1971). *Comparative Physiology of Respiratory Mechanisms*. Academic Press, New York and London.
248. WEBER, R. E. (1971). Oxygenational properties of vascular and coelomic haemoglobins from *Nephtys hombergii* (Polychaeta) and their functional significance. *Neth. J. Sea Res.*, **5**, 240–51.

Index

Page numbers in *italic* refer to figures or tables